WHO Technical Report Series
1016

WHO Expert Committee on Biological Standardization

Sixty-ninth report

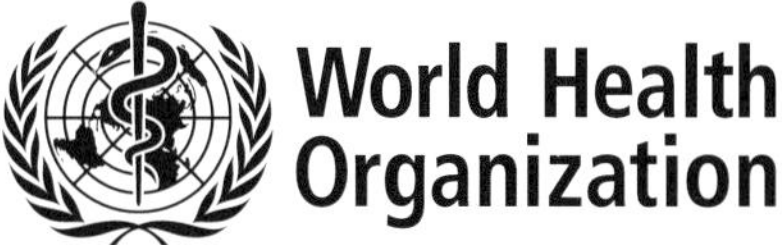

WHO Expert Committee on Biological Standardization: sixty-ninth report
(WHO Technical Report Series, No. 1016)
ISBN 9 789241 210256
ISSN 0512-3054

Contents

WHO Expert Committee on Biological Standardization
29 October to 2 November 2018

Committee members[1]

Dr C. Burns, National Institute for Biological Standards and Control, Potters Bar, the United Kingdom

Professor K. Cichutek, Paul-Ehrlich-Institut, Langen, Germany (*Chair*)

Dr M. Darko,[2] Food and Drugs Authority, Accra, Ghana

Dr J. Epstein, Center for Biologics Evaluation and Research, Food and Drug Administration, Silver Spring, MD, United States of America (the USA)

Dr S. Hindawi, Professor of Haematology & Transfusion Medicine, King Abdalaziz University, Jeddah, Saudi Arabia

Mrs T. Jivapaisarnpong, Lad Prao, Bangkok, Thailand (*Rapporteur for the plenary sessions and for the vaccines and biotherapeutics track*)

Dr H. Klein, National Institutes of Health, Bethesda, MD, the USA (*Vice-Chair*)

Dr C. Morris, National Institute for Biological Standards and Control, Potters Bar, the United Kingdom (*Rapporteur for the blood products and in vitro diagnostics track*)

Mr V.R. Reddy, South African National Blood Service, Weltevreden Park, South Africa

Dr P. Strengers, Sanquin, Amsterdam, Netherlands

Dr Y. Sohn, Seoul National University, Seoul, Republic of Korea

Dr J. Wang, National Institutes for Food and Drug Control, Beijing, China

Temporary Advisers

Ms A. Bonhomme,[2] Public Health Agency of Canada, Ottawa, Canada

Dr K. Chumakov, Center for Biologics Evaluation and Research, Food and Drug Administration, Bethesda, MD, the USA

Dr O.G. Engelhardt, National Institute for Biological Standards and Control, Potters Bar, the United Kingdom

Dr E. Griffiths, Kingston upon Thames, the United Kingdom (*Rapporteur for the plenary sessions and for the vaccines and biotherapeutics track*)

---

[1] The decisions of the Committee were taken in closed session with only members of the Committee present. Each Committee member had completed a Declaration of Interests form prior to the meeting. These were assessed by the WHO Secretariat and no declared interests were considered to be in conflict with full meeting participation.

[2] Unable to attend.

Dr G. Grohmann, University of Sydney, Sydney, Australia

Dr J.M. Katz,[3] Centers for Disease Control and Prevention, Atlanta, GA, the USA

Dr P. Kurki,[4] University of Helsinki, Helsinki, Finland

Dr J. Martin, National Institute for Biological Standards and Control, Potters Bar, the United Kingdom

Dr P. Minor, St Albans, the United Kingdom

Dr M. Powell,[4] Medicines and Healthcare Products Regulatory Agency, London, the United Kingdom

Dr J. Reinhardt, Paul-Ehrlich-Institut, Langen, Germany (*Rapporteur for the blood products and in vitro diagnostics track*)

Dr J. Southern, Representative of the South African Health Products Regulatory Authority, Simon's Town, South Africa

Dr Y. Sun, Paul-Ehrlich-Institut, Langen, Germany

Dr R. Thorpe, Welwyn, the United Kingdom

Dr A.L. Waddell, Stanley, the United Kingdom

Dr R. Webby, St. Jude Children's Research Hospital, Memphis, TN, the USA

Dr J. Weir, Center for Biologics Evaluation and Research, Food and Drug Administration, Silver Spring, MD, the USA

Dr T. Wu, Biologics and Genetic Therapies Directorate, Health Canada, Ottawa, Canada

Dr Q. Zhao, Xiamen University, Xiamen, China

State actors

Dr F. Agbanyo, Biologics and Genetic Therapies Directorate, Health Canada, Ottawa, Canada

Dr N. Almond, National Institute for Biological Standards and Control, Potters Bar, the United Kingdom

Dr P. Aprea, National Administration of Drugs, Food and Medical Technology, Buenos Aires, Argentina

Dr J. Boyle,[4] National Institute for Biological Standards and Control, Potters Bar, the United Kingdom

---

[3] Unable to attend.

[4] Participated via teleconference.

Dr H. Chan,[5] National Institute for Biological Standards and Control, Potters Bar, the United Kingdom

Dr H. Chun, Ministry of Food and Drug Safety, Chungcheongbuk-do, Republic of Korea

Dr B. Cowper,[5] National Institute for Biological Standards and Control, Potters Bar, the United Kingdom

Dr J. Ferguson,[5] National Institute for Biological Standards and Control, Potters Bar, the United Kingdom

Dr B. Fox,[5] National Institute for Biological Standards and Control, Potters Bar, the United Kingdom

Dr J. Fryer,[5] National Institute for Biological Standards and Control, Potters Bar, the United Kingdom

Dr I. Hamaguchi, National Institute of Infectious Diseases, Tokyo, Japan

Dr K. Han, Ministry of Food and Drug Safety, Chungcheongbuk-do, Republic of Korea

Dr R. Hawkins,[5] National Institute for Biological Standards and Control, Potters Bar, the United Kingdom

Dr A. Hilger, Paul-Ehrlich-Institut, Langen, Germany (*WHO Blood Regulators Network (BRN) Chair*)

Dr M.M. Ho,[5] National Institute for Biological Standards and Control, Potters Bar, the United Kingdom

Dr J. Hogwood,[5] National Institute for Biological Standards and Control, Potters Bar, the United Kingdom

Dr A. Hubbard,[5] National Institute for Biological Standards and Control, Potters Bar, the United Kingdom

Dr C.C. Ilonze, National Agency for Food and Drug Administration and Control, Lagos, Nigeria

Dr K. Ishii, National Institute of Infectious Diseases, Tokyo, Japan

Dr D. Kaslow,[5] Center for Vaccine Innovation and Access, Seattle, WA, the USA

Mr B.C. Kim, Ministry of Food and Drug Safety, Chungcheongbuk-do, Republic of Korea

Dr G. Mattiuzo,[5] National Institute for Biological Standards and Control, Potters Bar, the United Kingdom

Dr H. Meyer, Paul-Ehrlich-Institut, Langen, Germany

Dr M. Moore,[5] National Institute for Biological Standards and Control, Potters Bar, the United Kingdom

---

[5] Participated via teleconference.

Dr M. Nübling, Paul-Ehrlich-Institut, Langen, Germany

Dr M. Ochiai, National Institute of Infectious Diseases, Tokyo, Japan

Dr O. O'Shea,[6] National Institute for Biological Standards and Control, Potters Bar, the United Kingdom

Dr G. Prescott,[6] National Institute for Biological Standards and Control, Potters Bar, the United Kingdom

Dr C. Ranga, FDA Bhavan, New Delhi, India

Dr G. Raychaudhuri, Center for Biologics Evaluation and Research, Food and Drug Administration, Silver Spring, MD, the USA

Dr N. Rose, National Institute for Biological Standards and Control, Potters Bar, the United Kingdom

Dr M. Rosu-Myles, Biologics and Genetic Therapies Directorate, Health Canada, Ottawa, Canada

Dr P. Sanzone,[6] National Institute for Biological Standards and Control, Potters Bar, the United Kingdom

Dr L. de Jesus Saraiva,[6] National Institute for Biological Standards and Control, Potters Bar, the United Kingdom

Dr C. Schärer, Swiss Agency for Therapeutic Products, Bern, Switzerland

Dr G. Smith, Therapeutic Goods Administration, Woden, ACT, Australia

Dr P. Stickings, National Institute for Biological Standards and Control, Potters Bar, the United Kingdom

Dr C. Thelwell,[6] National Institute for Biological Standards and Control, Potters Bar, the United Kingdom

Dr A. Vasheghani, Food and Drug Organization, Tehran, the Islamic Republic of Iran

Dr D. Wilkinson,[6] National Institute for Biological Standards and Control, Potters Bar, the United Kingdom

Representation from non-state actors

Biotechnology Innovation Organization
Dr S. Ausborn, Roche, Basel, Switzerland

Coalition for Epidemic Preparedness Innovations
Dr J. Holst, Oslo, Norway

---

[6] Participated via teleconference.

Developing Countries Vaccine Manufacturers Network
Dr V. Paradkar, Biological E Ltd, Hyderabad, India

European Directorate for the Quality of Medicines & HealthCare
Dr K-H. Buchheit, Department of Biological Standardisation, OMCL Network & HealthCare, Strasbourg, France

Dr E. Charton, European Pharmacopoeia Department, Strasbourg, France

Dr M. Wierer, Department of Biological Standardisation, OMCL Network & HealthCare, Strasbourg, France

International Federation of Pharmaceutical Manufacturers & Associations
Dr M. Gencoglu, Geneva, Switzerland

International Generic and Biosimilar Medicines Association
Dr I. Schwarzenberger, Sandoz

Pharmaceutical and Medical Device Regulatory Science Society of Japan (formerly Society of Japanese Pharmacopoeia)
Dr Y. Nakagawa, Osaka, Japan

Plasma Protein Therapeutics Association
Dr D. Misztela, Brussels, Belgium

WHO Secretariat
Regional Office
WHO Regional Office for the Americas – Dr M-L. Pombo

WHO Regional Office for the Eastern Mediterranean – Dr H. Langar

Headquarters
Dr F. Lery, Coordinator, TSN/EMP *(Lead (a.i.) for the blood products and in vitro diagnostics track)*

Dr I. Knezevic, TSN/EMP *(Secretary to the Committee; Lead for the vaccines and biotherapeutics track)*

Ms S. Jenner, TSN/EMP

Dr H-N. Kang, TSN/EMP

Dr D. Lei, TSN/EMP

Dr T. Zhou, TSN/EMP

Abbreviations

Ab	antibody
AfSBT	African Society for Blood Transfusion
Ag	antigen
BRN	WHO Blood Regulators Network
CBER	Center for Biologics Evaluation and Research
CCHF	Crimean-Congo haemorrhagic fever
CEPI	Coalition for Epidemic Preparedness Innovations
cfDNA	circulating cell-free DNA
CHIM	controlled human infection model
CRF	circulating recombinant form
ctDNA	circulating cell-free tumour DNA
CVV	candidate vaccine virus
D-Ag	D-Antigen
DNA	deoxyribonucleic acid
ECSPP	WHO Expert Committee on Specifications for Pharmaceutical Preparations
EDL	WHO Model List of Essential In Vitro Diagnostics
EDQM	European Directorate for the Quality of Medicines & HealthCare
ELISA	enzyme-linked immunosorbent assay
EML	WHO Model List of Essential Medicines
ERL	WHO essential regulatory laboratory
EUAL	WHO emergency use assessment and listing (procedure)
EV	enterovirus
FFPE	formalin-fixed paraffin-embedded
fPSA	free prostate specific antigen
FV:Ag	blood coagulation factor V antigen
FV:C	blood coagulation factor V clotting activity
FXa	activated blood coagulation factor X

WHO Technical Report Series, No. 1016, 2019

GAPIII	WHO Global Action Plan to minimize poliovirus facility-associated risk after type-specific eradication of wild polioviruses and sequential cessation of oral polio vaccine use
GBT	Global Benchmarking Tool
GCV	geometric coefficient of variation
GISRS	WHO Global Influenza Surveillance and Response System
GMP	good manufacturing practice(s)
GPIb	glycoprotein Ib
HA	haemagglutinin
HAdV	human adenovirus
HEV	hepatitis E virus
HIV	human immunodeficiency virus
HPAEC-PAD	high-performance anion exchange chromatography with pulsed amperometric detection
HPAI	highly pathogenic avian influenza
HPLC	high-performance liquid chromatography
HPV	human papillomavirus
ICDRA	International Conference of Drug Regulatory Authorities
IDMS	isotope-dilution mass spectrometry
IFU	instructions for use
IGF-I	insulin-like growth factor-I
IgG	immunoglobulin G
IgM	immunoglobulin M
INN	international nonproprietary name(s)
IPV	inactivated poliomyelitis vaccine
ISTH	International Society on Thrombosis and Haemostasis
IU	International Unit(s)
IVD	in vitro diagnostic
IVPP	influenza viruses with pandemic potential
LMIC	low- and middle-income countries

mAb	monoclonal antibody
MAPREC	mutant analysis by polymerase chain reaction and restriction enzyme cleavage
MCB	master cell bank
MERS-CoV	Middle East respiratory syndrome coronavirus
MSC	mesenchymal stromal cell
MSI	microsatellite instability
NAT	nucleic acid amplification technique
NCL	national control laboratory
NGS	next-generation sequencing
NIBSC	National Institute for Biological Standards and Control
NIFDC	National Institutes for Food and Drug Control
NIH	National Institutes of Health
NRA	national regulatory authority
OPV	oral poliomyelitis vaccine
PCR	polymerase chain reaction
PDMP	plasma-derived medicinal product
PDVAC	WHO Product Development for Vaccines Advisory Committee
PEI	Paul-Ehrlich-Institut
PHE	public health emergency
PIK3	phosphatidylinositol-4,5-bisphosphate 3-kinase
PIK3CA	phosphatidylinositol-4,5-bisphosphate 3-kinase catalytic subunit alpha (gene)
PLS	primary liquid standard
PSA	prostate specific antigen
qNMR	quantitative nuclear magnetic resonance
RCB	reference cell bank
RNA	ribonucleic acid
RSV	respiratory syncytial virus
SAGE	Strategic Advisory Group of Experts (on Immunization)

SAGE IVD	Strategic Advisory Group of Experts on In Vitro Diagnostics
SBP	similar biotherapeutic product
SDU	Sabin D-Ag Unit(s)
SE–HPLC	size-exclusion high-performance liquid chromatography
sIPV	Sabin inactivated poliomyelitis vaccine
SRA	stringent regulatory authority
SRD	single radial immunodiffusion (assay)
TB	tuberculosis
TPO	thyroid peroxidase
UHC	universal health coverage
URF	unique recombinant form
US FDA	United States Food and Drug Administration
VLP	virus-like particle
VWF	Von Willebrand factor
WHOCC	WHO collaborating centre
WLA	WHO-listed authority

1. Introduction

The WHO Expert Committee on Biological Standardization met in Geneva from 29 October to 2 November 2018. The meeting was opened on behalf of the Director-General of WHO by Dr Soumya Swaminathan, Deputy Director-General for Programmes. Dr Swaminathan welcomed the Committee, meeting participants and observers, and reminded them that this was the longest serving WHO expert committee and was very much valued by WHO for its contribution to global public health over many years. It was further recognized that recent years had seen a rapid expansion of the biologicals field, leading to the development of novel biotherapeutic products, vaccines, cellular therapies and in vitro diagnostics (IVDs). This had resulted in an ever greater demand for biological standardization efforts.

The Committee was reminded that one of the cornerstones of WHO efforts to advance towards universal health coverage (UHC) is equitable access to safe, quality and affordable medical products – an area in which the setting of global standards will be essential. Dr Swaminathan acknowledged the contribution made by national regulatory authorities (NRAs) in meeting the need for affordable biologicals of known quality and efficacy, and highlighted the key role of international norms and standards in facilitating regulatory convergence.

The Committee was informed that the WHO prequalification programme was also expanding – again increasing demand for appropriate international standards. There was also a growing need for standards to support the measures being taken against the priority pathogens identified in the WHO Blueprint for Research and Development: Responding to Public Health Emergencies of International Concern (WHO R&D Blueprint) which was designed to improve readiness against future health emergencies due to infectious agents. Biological products, such as IVDs and vaccines are among the most promising interventions for dealing with such infections and the engagement of the Committee together with other organizations will be of the utmost importance.

Dr Swaminathan recognized that the Committee had a very heavy agenda and much to deal with in one week. To manage this agenda it would be necessary to meet not only in plenary sessions but also in two parallel tracks. As in previous years, one track would focus on vaccines and biotherapeutics and the other on blood products and IVDs. It was recognized that having two tracks running in parallel places a heavy burden on the meeting chairs and rapporteurs. On behalf of WHO, Dr Swaminathan expressed her thanks to the Committee, to the WHO collaborating centres (WHOCCs) and to all the experts, institutions and professional societies working in this area, all of whose efforts provide vital support to WHO programmes working in global public health and to NRAs worldwide.

Dr Ivana Knezevic, Secretary to the Committee, thanked Dr Swaminathan for her opening remarks and announced the details of the working arrangements for the present meeting which differed in certain respects from previous meetings. Committee members, regulatory authority representatives and subject matter experts from governmental organizations would participate in the meeting from 29 October to 1 November 2018. This section of the meeting would end following the morning session of 1 November, with the chairs and rapporteurs meeting in the afternoon to draft an early version of the Committee report. An open information-sharing session involving all participants, including non-state actors, would be held on 29 October. Final decisions on the adoption of written standards and the establishment of measurement standards would be made by the Committee members during a closed session held on 2 November.

Dr Knezevic then moved on to the election of the meeting officials. In the absence of dissent, Professor Klaus Cichutek was elected as Chair and Dr Elwyn Griffiths and Mrs Teeranart Jivapaisarnpong as Rapporteurs for the plenary sessions and for the vaccines and biotherapeutics track. Dr Harvey Klein was elected as Chair and Dr Clare Morris and Dr Jens Reinhardt as Rapporteurs for the blood products and in vitro diagnostics track. Dr Klein was also elected as Vice-Chair for the plenary sessions of the Committee.

Dr Knezevic introduced each of the members of the Committee and then presented the declarations of interests that had been made by them and by WHO temporary advisers and participants. After evaluation, WHO had concluded that none of the declarations made constituted a significant conflict of interest and that the individuals concerned would be allowed to participate fully in the meeting. Committee members and WHO temporary advisers were reminded that they acted in their own personal capacities as experts and not as representatives of their own organizations or countries.

Following participant introductions, the Committee adopted the proposed agenda and timetable (WHO/BS/2018.2353).

2. General

 Current directions

 Strategic directions in the regulation of medicines and other health technologies: WHO priorities

Dr Francois-Xavier Lery presented an overview of strategic directions and WHO priorities in the area of biologicals. Under the guidance of the new Director-General, the WHO thirteenth general programme of work 2019–2023 aims to build healthier populations, deal with health emergencies and promote UHC. Achieving these aims will require ensuring greater access to quality-assured health products through effective and efficient regulatory systems. This will involve addressing issues such as the efficacy and safety of medicines, their quality assurance and their affordability. WHO regulatory programmes would continue to work closely together to deliver coordinated support to national regulators, with a strong focus placed on outcomes while at the same time maintaining required standards.

A 5-year Strategic Plan (2019–2023) has now been developed to adapt the WHO thirteenth general programme of work to country needs and situations based on four priority areas:

- Strengthening country and regional regulatory systems, including through the promotion of regulatory reliance and collaboration, as an integral part of the drive towards UHC.

- Improving regulatory preparedness for public health emergencies (PHEs), including medicine shortages. The WHO emergency use assessment and listing (EUAL) procedure had been introduced following the 2014 Ebola outbreaks in Africa in order to expedite the availability of medical products needed during a public health emergency of international concern (PHEIC). As of June 2018, nine diagnostic tests had been evaluated (seven for Ebola virus and two for Zika virus) along with three applications for Ebola vaccines.

- Maintaining and expanding WHO prequalification and product risk assessment to promote healthier populations. A WHO pilot procedure for the prequalification of biotherapeutic products or their corresponding similar biotherapeutic products (SBPs) was now under way focusing on rituximab and trastuzumab (see section 2.4.6).

- Optimizing the impact of WHO regulatory support activities.

The Committee was then informed that WHO will replace the term "stringent regulatory authority (SRA)" with "WHO-listed authority (WLA)". The concept of an SRA had originally been based on membership of the International Council for Harmonisation of Technical Requirements for Pharmaceuticals for Human Use and had been developed to promote reliance and guide procurement decisions. Despite the term being widely used in WHO written standards there was a growing view that such a change in terminology was needed. Currently recognized SRAs will be regarded as WLAs, with additional NRAs designated as such based on the WHO Global Benchmarking Tool (GBT) plus completion of a confidence-building process and a broader consultation process.

The Committee was further informed that monitoring of the impact of WHO activities on regulation and on access to medicines and health products was being reinforced. Impact monitoring activities, including an impact assessment of the prequalification procedure sponsored by UNITAID, are now under way. These have already resulted in a number of useful recommendations in relation to WHO operational and communications activities in this area. In the case of norms and standards, implementation rates by NRAs and manufacturers have increased following workshops, training and the provision of WHO questions-and-answers resources.

Dr Lery concluded by pointing out that the work of the Committee was a fundamental enabler of many WHO normative and regulatory activities, with strong links to other WHO activities such as the WHO Strategic Advisory Group of Experts (SAGE) on Immunization. The efforts of the Committee and of the WHO networks of collaborating centres in the standardization and regulatory evaluation of medicines and other health technologies were crucial in enabling WHO to adapt to the evolving environment of emerging diseases and advanced therapies. Dr Lery affirmed that WHO remained committed to supporting the implementation of the normative guidance developed by the Committee and to ensuring the uptake and implementation of the measurement standards established by it. Dr Lery thanked the Committee for its considerable efforts in this field.

The Committee thanked Dr Lery for his useful overview of current and planned WHO regulatory activities, and for highlighting the key role played by the Committee. The Committee provided a number of comments on the move to replace the concept of an SRA with a WLA based on the WHO GBT. The implementation of this approach would require sufficient assurance of the regulatory competency and experience of WLAs, especially with regard to highly sophisticated novel biological products, such as SBPs and cellular therapies. It was noted that WHO Guidelines on good regulatory and reliance practices were under development and there would thus be an opportunity to address these issues.

2.1.2 Vaccines and biotherapeutics: recent and planned activities in biological standardization

Dr Knezevic reported on recent and planned WHO activities in relation to the biological standardization and regulatory evaluation of vaccines and biotherapeutics. Historically, a total of 93 written standards (primarily WHO Recommendations and WHO Guidelines) had been recommended for adoption by the Committee. In addition, a large number of measurement standards (primarily WHO international standards and WHO international reference reagents) had been established and were essential for the development, licensing and ongoing lot release of biological medicines. Measurement standards established between 2013 and 2017 included several antibody standards. Such standards were particularly important in standardizing the measurement of antibody responses to vaccines during clinical development and in supporting ongoing regulatory oversight. However, some vaccine developers remained unfamiliar with the need for assay standardization, and with the role of biological standards in supporting the development of safe and effective products. Dr Knezevic emphasized the importance of continuing to promote the use of antibody and other standards even though it was not always obvious how best to do this. The work of the WHO network of collaborating centres on standardization and regulatory evaluation of vaccines provided invaluable support in this respect (see section 2.2.2).

In 2016 and 2017 the Committee had recommended the adoption of a total of four new WHO written standards for vaccines and one revised document. At the present meeting, new WHO Recommendations on hepatitis E vaccines (see section 3.4.1) and two revised WHO Guidelines dealing with the safe production of influenza and poliomyelitis vaccines were to be considered for adoption (see sections 3.4.2 and 3.4.3 respectively). In addition, following the recent adoption of two new WHO Guidelines on biotherapeutic products, a WHO questions-and-answers document based on the current WHO Guidelines on evaluation of similar biotherapeutic products (SBPs) would also be considered for adoption at the present meeting (see section 3.2.1). New or revised written standards for respiratory syncytial virus (RSV) vaccines, meningitis B vaccines, DNA vaccines, inactivated poliomyelitis vaccine (IPV) and EV71 vaccines were scheduled for consideration by the Committee in 2019–2020. Looking forward, new WHO Guidelines on insulin have been proposed, along with the revision of the WHO Recommendations for the preparation, characterization and establishment of international and other biological reference standards (see section 3.1.1).

Dr Knezevic indicated that in view of current resources it was difficult to prioritize these different projects since each entailed a considerable workload. For example, the development of RSV vaccines is progressing rapidly and the

WHO Guidelines to assure their quality, safety and efficacy were discussed at a consultation in September 2018. Further revision and public consultation will now be required prior to submission to the Committee in 2019. In addition, there are plans for a workshop in 2019 on the use of measurement standards for antibodies to RSV – the First WHO International Standard for antiserum to respiratory syncytial virus having been established by the Committee in 2017. The suitability of this standard for monoclonal antibody (mAb) competition assays was currently being assessed and there may be a need for additional WHO international standards. The question of training and implementation workshops in relation to the use of such standards would then also need to be considered.

The Committee was informed that the development of nucleic acid based vaccines was now progressing rapidly following earlier setbacks. WHO was monitoring the situation and had held a consultation on developments in this area in February 2018. Therapeutic and prophylactic DNA vaccines are considered to be the most likely products to reach licensure first, followed by RNA vaccines. Regulators had highlighted the need to update the 2007 WHO Guidelines for assuring the quality and nonclinical safety evaluation of DNA vaccines with regard to prophylaxis and therapy. Although there was less need at present for the development of guidance on RNA vaccines, an early "points to consider" document may be required. Dr Knezevic also reported on the considerable efforts being made to develop Zika vaccines and on the need for their standardization (see section 8.1.1). A joint WHO/National Institutes of Health consultation on Zika vaccines had been held in March 2018 to identify strategies for demonstrating Zika vaccine effectiveness in the context of waning disease incidence.

Dr Knezevic then reported on the WHO 2016–2018 programme of implementation workshops on WHO Recommendations and Guidelines. WHO Recommendations and Guidelines are considered to be excellent tools for promoting regulatory convergence as well as important educational and training tools for improving NRA expertise, and are thus central to facilitating access to biologicals of appropriate quality, safety and efficacy. During the course of 2016–2018, numerous implementation workshops had been held covering a wide range of WHO written standards, including those on good manufacturing practices (GMP), typhoid conjugate vaccines and biotherapeutics including SBPs. These workshops involved the use of case studies as these are considered to be an extremely useful training resource for NRAs, with several such case studies from previous workshops having also been published in the scientific press. The 2018 International Conference of Drug Regulatory Authorities (ICDRA) had recommended that WHO should continue organizing implementation workshops to accelerate the use of the WHO Guidelines on evaluation of similar biotherapeutic products (SBPs) by Member States.

ICDRA had further recommended that these workshops should focus more on analytical comparability than on comparability in clinical data, and that the importance of regulatory oversight throughout the entire life-cycle of SBPs should be emphasized. Dr Knezevic concluded by highlighting a number of opportunities and challenges in promoting regulatory convergence. Although significant challenges remain, there are also many international and regional regulatory, industry and other networks and organizations working in this area, with corresponding opportunities to update the scientific community on the development of WHO standards and to collaborate in training and other initiatives to promote their implementation.

The Committee thanked Dr Knezevic for her report and expressed support for the proposed initiatives. However, some reservations remained concerning the perceived urgency to update the WHO Guidelines for assuring the quality and nonclinical safety evaluation of DNA vaccines. Despite significant developments in this area, no DNA vaccine had yet been licensed for human use and characterization of the immune responses had not yet been defined. Nevertheless, the scaling-up of manufacture to produce useful quantities of good quality vaccine was an issue and updated guidance on this could be helpful. Conflicting views were also expressed on the status of RNA vaccines and on the significance of current developments. The Committee concluded that WHO should continue to monitor the development of such vaccines. The Committee also drew attention to the WHO guidance document on human challenge trials for vaccine development: regulatory considerations. Although the document addressed most of the key issues, additional care would be needed in relation to ethical perspectives, and consideration given to whether data from such studies can be accepted or not in all jurisdictions. The development of guidance on how to select and develop animal models might also be of value.

2.1.3 Blood products and in vitro diagnostics: recent and planned activities in biological standardization

Dr Lery informed the Committee that following the departure of Dr Micha Nübling (WHO Lead for the blood products and in vitro diagnostics track) Dr Yuyun Maryuningsih would shortly be appointed to this role for future meetings of the Committee. Dr Lery then presented an overview of recent and planned activities in the areas of blood products and IVDs with a focus on: (a) blood regulation; (b) the impact of emerging infections on the blood supply; (c) the work of the WHO network of collaborating centres for blood products and in vitro diagnostics; (d) snake envenoming; and (e) health emergencies.

Dr Lery first outlined the recent efforts made by WHO and partner organizations that had resulted in the establishment of the African Blood Regulators Forum under the umbrella of the African Medicines Regulatory

Harmonization initiative. An update was provided on the development of a multi-criteria decision analysis tool intended to guide regulatory decision-making on the safety of the blood supply in the context of emerging infections.

Dr Lery then reported on the work of the WHO network of collaborating centres for blood products and in vitro diagnostics during 2018. There was agreement that updating the current WHO Recommendations for the preparation, characterization and establishment of international and other biological reference standards would be beneficial (see section 3.1.1) particularly given its present insufficient coverage of the diagnostics field. It had further been agreed that two new WHO measurement standards for blood products were ready for submission to the Committee for possible establishment, along with three new projects for endorsement. In addition, eight new measurement standards for IVDs were to be submitted for possible establishment and 12 new projects proposed for endorsement.

Discussions had also been held between IVD manufacturers, donors, academic experts and the WHO network of collaborating centres for blood products and in vitro diagnostics on the need to develop standards for IVDs and vaccine candidates for use during PHEs. Related developments in this area included the establishment of a biological standardization and assays working group by the recently launched Coalition for Epidemic Preparedness Innovations (CEPI). A report on the development of proposed WHO international standards for emerging and re-emerging viruses with epidemic potential and on the collaborative efforts now under way in this area is presented below in section 8.2.2.

Efforts to address snake envenoming were also under way but numerous challenges remain, for example in developing specific standards for different snake species in different parts of the world and in standardizing antivenom production processes. The assessing of antivenoms for listing on the WHO website and potential future WHO prequalification had previously been reported on and was continuing (see section 5.2.3).

The Committee thanked Dr Lery for his report and looked forward to being updated on progress in these areas.

2.1.4   WHO comprehensive plan for the blood programme

Dr Lery presented an overview of the WHO programme to advance universal access to quality and safe blood and blood components for transfusion and to plasma-derived medicinal products (PDMPs). Blood and blood products play an essential role in promoting and safeguarding human health but a number of key global challenges remain. In 2016, data from the WHO Global Database on Blood Safety had been used as the basis of the *WHO Global status report on blood safety and availability*.

Dr Lery pointed out that the first priority for national blood regulation was the establishment of specific legislation that incorporated blood and blood products into law. Only then could a well-functioning blood regulatory system be established and strengthened through capacity-building, training and other activities. At present, many countries still relied on approaches based on self-regulation by blood establishments. Despite the technical know-how of blood establishments, this is not considered to be a desirable situation as only independent regulatory oversight can assure product safety. In addition, regulatory oversight will help to prevent the perception of a conflict of interests, for example when a commercially relevant product needs to be withdrawn from the market due to potential safety issues. Other key challenges include suboptimal clinical practices in blood product handling, barriers to achieving universal access to blood and blood products, and the need to improve haemovigilance.

Dr Lery outlined potential approaches for improving the integration and coordination of various WHO blood programme activities – for example, WHO prequalification of diagnostic tests crucial in blood-transfusion safety and WHO efforts to strengthen regulatory systems – with the work of the BRN and the blood and IVD track of the Committee. It was proposed that an annual forum be established to strengthen communication between the various groups, address stakeholders and review WHO guideline needs and implementation status.

During discussion it was highlighted that the issue of blood and blood products was not always seen as a high priority by countries and that continued advocacy was needed. The Committee also provided a number of recommendations for improving evaluation of the impact of WHO activities. The use of interim and other metrics, for example changes in national guidelines and legislation directly resulting from WHO activities, might usefully be incorporated into impact evaluation frameworks. The question was asked of whether the declaration of blood and blood products as essential medicines by the World Health Assembly had beneficially impacted on activities in this area. This was indeed viewed as a positive step, with numerous requests having been made by many countries to experienced regulatory authorities in relation to blood regulation. Discussion of this topic at the 2016 ICDRA meeting also reflected increased awareness of the relevance of blood regulation. It was pointed out however that while awareness of the GMP requirements of blood and blood components had increased, these are very different from conventional pharmaceutical products and further clarification of this may be needed.

The Committee expressed appreciation for the comprehensive plan presented for the WHO blood programme. The Committee also agreed to review draft versions of the plan and to provide comments in relation to the scope of planned activities and the addressing of gaps.

2.2 Reports

2.2.1 Report from the WHO Blood Regulators Network

Dr Anneliese Hilger, Chair of the BRN, reported on the activities of the network in 2017–2018. The Committee was reminded that the objectives of BRN were to promote the science-based convergence of regulatory policy, foster international consensus on regulatory approaches, provide scientific assessments of current and emerging threats and propose solutions to specific issues – particularly emerging public health challenges. BRN had held four teleconferences during 2018 following a face-to-face meeting in October 2017, with another such meeting scheduled in the coming days. Agenda items for this upcoming meeting included finalization of the maturity levels of blood indicators, issues in relation to hepatitis E virus (HEV), and the setting of the BRN workplan for 2018–2019 – including the continuation of its work with WHO regional offices. Existing BRN position papers would also be reviewed at this meeting, along with a request from the International Society of Blood Transfusion Working Party on Transfusion Transmitted Infectious Diseases for a BRN statement on the use of virus inactivated cryoprecipitates in low-resource settings.

In its 2017–2018 workplan BRN had aimed to strengthen stakeholder involvement in the work of the WHO regional offices. Meetings had been held with the WHO Regional Office for Africa and with the WHO Regional Office for the Eastern Mediterranean. A draft model blood legislation prepared by the WHO Regional Office for the Eastern Mediterranean had been reviewed. Contact was now being made with the WHO Regional Office for the Western Pacific. BRN had also participated in a WHO workshop in Cameroon and had held a workshop on the safety of blood and blood products at the 2018 ICDRA meeting in Dublin. Among the ICDRA workshop recommendations was that WHO Member States should be encouraged to take steps to establish or strengthen their national haemovigilance systems in accordance with the WHO Guidelines on estimation of residual risk of HIV, HBV or HCV infections via cellular blood components and plasma. In particular, WHO Member States were encouraged to engage in both internal and external assessments of their national haemovigilance systems using the WHO GBT and incorporating the WHO assessment criteria for national regulatory systems. Workshop participants also called on WHO to support the establishment of national haemovigilance systems in Member States through the facilitation of educational and training opportunities at regional level.

The Committee thanked Dr Hilger for her report and acknowledged the support that BRN provides to the work of WHO.

2.2.2 Report from the WHO network of collaborating centres on standardization and regulatory evaluation of vaccines

Dr Paul Stickings and Dr Junzhi Wang reported on the fourth meeting of the network held in September 2018 at the new facilities of the National Institutes for Food and Drug Control (NIFDC) in Beijing. Among the topics discussed in depth at the meeting were: (a) the proposed development of procedures for the pre-review of WHO measurement standards by the collaborating centres to support the work of the Committee; (b) the proposed update of the WHO Recommendations for the preparation, characterization and establishment of international and other biological reference standards (see section 3.1.1); (c) the development of standards for priority pathogens identified as potential causes of future PHEs; and (d) the replacement of the WHO Vero reference cell bank 10-87. Updates on the activities of all the network members had also been provided at the meeting.

In relation to the proposal that the network might usefully pre-review selected WHO measurement standards in order to expedite the Committee review processes, meeting participants had felt that the resources required to implement this could not be justified given a lack of clarity surrounding the degree to which this might be beneficial to the Committee. Nevertheless, it was agreed that the early engagement of the network may be valuable when new projects are proposed – a situation that already exists for proposed new projects in the areas of blood products and IVDs. It was suggested that WHO might consider organizing an annual meeting of the network early each year at which proposals for new projects could be reviewed. The aim would be to increase awareness of new proposals among the collaborating centres and to increase participation in the collaborative studies – along with other potential contributions, such as the provision of study samples. This would require the earlier submission of proposals for new work to WHO and the sharing of this information among all interested groups.

Consensus had also been reached during the network meeting on the need to revise the current WHO Recommendations on international and other biological reference standards. It was further suggested that consideration be given to creating two different documents – one for collaborating centres focused on the development of WHO international standards and the other for end users on the principles of biological standardization, particularly in relation to the calibration of secondary standards and assays. The development of the second document was considered to be the more pressing and could potentially be developed as a manual or scientific paper rather than as a formal annex to the report of the Committee. The holding of a consultation or workshop might also allow for improved understanding of the issues to be addressed and the required content of any new document intended for end users. It was envisaged that the scope of any such meeting would encompass reference materials for diagnostics, biotherapeutic products and vaccines, and would take into account the needs of the WHO prequalification programme.

The development of standards for priority pathogens was also extensively discussed at the network meeting as these are considered to be a high priority. Challenges and complications identified in this area include ethical issues related to the sourcing of patient materials, political factors involved in obtaining access to biological samples, biosafety issues and linked export/import hurdles. Such challenges had already increased the workload of the National Institute for Biological Standards and Control (NIBSC) and suggestions were made as to possible ways of addressing them. These included making a list of BSL4 facilities available in or to the collaborating centres, early communication between centres regarding the exporting/importing of study samples and the reaching of high-level pre-agreements – potentially facilitated by WHO – on the provision of materials for use in collaborative studies and as standards. It was suggested that the procedures used for pandemic influenza might provide a useful model to follow.

The Committee was also informed that discussions had taken place on the nearing depletion of the WHO Vero reference cell bank 10-87. Ideally, any replacement would need to be produced in a GMP-compliant facility. The very high level of demand for this cell line from manufacturers in China was noted and the collaborating centres had speculated on the possibility of establishing a national cell bank in China to meet this demand. Although this was technically possible the production of the cell bank would not be produced under full GMP and consideration would need to be given to the best way of addressing this issue (see section 3.1.2).

The Committee thanked Dr Stickings and Dr Wang for their report and noted the comments and suggestions made – some of which would be discussed further during the current meeting. The Committee expressed its support for the proposal to hold an annual meeting at which new projects could be reviewed, and recommended the joint participation of WHOCCs working in the areas of vaccines, blood products and IVDs in order to improve coordination between the two tracks of Committee meetings. The need to prioritize the development of guidance for end users of WHO international standards prior to updating the current WHO Recommendations was noted but there was less support expressed for publishing such guidance outside the WHO Technical Report Series in which the report of the Committee appears. Publishing WHO guidance on the development of international standards and the calibrating of secondary standards in the WHO Technical Report Series would ensure that the process for setting WHO international standards and other measurement standards remained clear and transparent. The Committee further noted that there was currently no direct link between the collaborating centres and the priority pathogen activities of WHO and other partners, such as CEPI. The Committee highlighted the crucial importance of establishing good links between all such partners to minimize potential overlap and ensure the coordinated implementation of vaccine and companion diagnostics projects in this area (see section 8.2.2).

2.3 Feedback from custodian laboratories

2.3.1 Developments and scientific issues highlighted by custodians of WHO biological reference preparations

The Committee was informed of recent developments and issues identified by the following custodians of WHO biological reference preparations.

National Institute for Biological Standards and Control (NIBSC), Potters Bar, the United Kingdom

Dr Stickings presented his report on behalf of the Director of NIBSC, Dr Christian Schneider, who was unable to attend. The Committee was informed that NIBSC currently holds 368 different WHO standards all of which are listed in the WHO catalogue. During the 2017–2018 reporting period, WHO standards were distributed to over 1000 recipients in 85 countries, with around 95% of all such standards held at NIBSC having been distributed to at least one recipient since the start of 2018. Dr Stickings noted that different WHO standards were used at different rates, reflecting not only the number of users of a specific standard but also how that standard was being used. A proportion of WHO international standards are expected to be used in very low amounts, while several are now very old and are hardly needed anymore. At the same time, the availability of a new WHO international standard does not guarantee that it will be adopted in practice – a problem primarily observed in the diagnostics field, but also in the development of vaccines against emerging diseases. For example, the use of Ebola standards was considered to be of high importance at the time of the 2014 outbreaks but assays were apparently not being calibrated against the First WHO International Reference Reagent for Ebola virus antibodies. Part of the problem is thought to be the routine use of SI units, particularly in the diagnostics field, as opposed to the International Units (IU) used for many WHO international standards. It was felt that more should perhaps be done to highlight this issue.

NIBSC also considered that more effort should be given to promoting the availability and appropriate use of WHO international standards. Various suggestions had been made as to how this might be done, including through publications and implementation workshops. It was acknowledged that some efforts would require significantly more resources than others, with some of the more routine applications perhaps being promoted through website and social media communications. NIBSC was actively working in this area and was keen to work with WHO and others in maximizing the impact of these international standards.

The Committee was reminded that NIBSC has a strategic objective to support innovation and the standardization of cellular and gene therapies (see section 3.3.1). Dr Stickings noted that several standards had already been established in this area and more would be proposed in the near future. The development of such standards is underpinned by assay development and by a research programme in the fields of cellular and gene therapies, and personalized and precision medicines, both of which are growing activity areas.

The Committee thanked Dr Stickings for his report. Agreement was expressed that more should be done to encourage the developers and end users of assays to use the WHO IU/ml unitage rather than SI unitage. The Committee also acknowledged the existence of some very old standards held at the NIBSC but also cautioned against their immediate disposal as it was possible they may still be needed on occasion. However, it was also recommended that consideration should be given to drawing up a list of rarely used or never used standards for consideration by the Committee and possible disestablishment.

European Directorate for the Quality of Medicines & HealthCare (EDQM), Strasbourg, France

Dr Karl-Heinz Buchheit reported on a number of recent EDQM activities in the area of international standards for antibiotics, and on the activities of the EDQM biological standardisation programme, in which WHO has Observer status. Dr Buchheit reminded the Committee that EDQM is the custodian centre for international standards for antibiotics – a responsibility it assumed from the NIBSC in 2006. Twenty three international standards for old antibiotics are currently available, eight of which are on the WHO Model List of Essential Medicines (EML). These international standards are indispensable in the calibration of regional and in-house standards. With the exception of erythromycin (see section 4.1.1) there was no requirement for any replacement antibiotic standards this year, and no issues had been identified since the last meeting of the Committee.

Dr Buchheit then turned to the recent activities of the biological standardisation programme, the goals of which are: (a) to establish European Pharmacopoeia biological reference preparations; (b) to standardize test methods for the quality control of biologicals; (c) to elaborate alternative test methods in order to further the application of the 3Rs principles (Replacement, Reduction, Refinement) regarding the use of animals in research; and (d) to promote international harmonization in the field of biologicals through collaboration with WHO and other partners. Current projects of particular interest to the

Committee include the potential replacement with serological assays of the current in vivo assays used for the potency testing of rabies vaccines and whole cell pertussis vaccines.

In the case of rabies vaccines, the Committee was informed that a G-protein-based enzyme-linked immunosorbent assay (ELISA) for non-adjuvanted rabies vaccines for human use had been developed and evaluated. This assay was now being promoted by the European Partnership for Alternative Approaches to Animal Testing as a potential replacement for the current in vivo assay. The assay has been shown to be suitable for all European as well as a number of non-European rabies vaccines (different strains) and can detect sub-potent vaccines. The good quality mAbs needed for the assay were now commercially available and reasonably priced and a collaborative study to assess the feasibility of the method in routine testing (and in the testing of marketed products) was expected to be undertaken in 2019.

The possible replacement of the Kendrick test for evaluating the potency of whole cell pertussis vaccines had also been carefully studied by EDQM. The in vivo test has been criticized both for its very poor reproducibility and for the extreme distress it causes to test animals. The alternative assay under evaluation involves the immunization of guinea-pigs or mice and subsequent preparation of serum samples after a stipulated time for testing by ELISA. The results of a collaborative study involving eight laboratories indicated that the ELISA accurately discriminated between compliant and non-compliant products, and ranked the tested vaccines similarly to the Kendrick test. Due to the high variability of Kendrick test results and differences in the nature of the parameter measured in the two tests a direct correlation with Kendrick values had not being possible. EDQM had concluded that the ELISA was suitable for use in routine consistency testing of whole cell pertussis vaccines following product-specific validation, and would propose its inclusion as an alternative to the Kendrick test in the European Pharmacopoeia. This information was now being presented to the Committee for its consideration in the context of the WHO Recommendations for whole cell pertussis vaccine.

The Committee thanked Dr Buchheit for his report and noted the proposal to include the serological assay for the potency testing of whole cell pertussis vaccines in the European Pharmacopoeia as a consistency test. The replacement of the in vivo challenge potency assay in mice (the so-called "Kendrick test") had long been considered and had previously been discussed by the Committee. At that time it was felt that the serological approaches could not be considered as validated alternatives and they were therefore not included in the revised WHO Recommendations for whole cell pertussis vaccine. However, the revised Recommendations do include the strong recommendation from EDQM that manufacturers and control laboratories use validated humane end-points in mouse protection tests. The Committee agreed that the new data reported at this meeting should be reviewed in more detail. It was noted however that if the serological test were to be used for routine consistency testing following product-specific validation then the issue would arise of how to retain expertise in conducting the in vivo Kendrick test for possible occasional use – an issue common to other vaccines.

Paul-Ehrlich-Institut (PEI), Langen, Germany

Dr Heidi Meyer reported on the activities of PEI over the past year and on a number of scientific issues of interest. Dr Meyer provided an update on the progress made in two projects previously endorsed by the Committee – namely, the development of a WHO reference material for anti-chikungunya virus immunoglobulin M (IgM) and immunoglobulin G (IgG) and a WHO reference panel for HEV antibodies. PEI had participated in a 2018 CEPI workshop on chikungunya virus in New Delhi at which the main correlates of protection were agreed to be neutralizing antibodies. However, due to high variability between the assays used to measure such antibodies there was a recognized need for assay standardization efforts. PEI had therefore collected and characterized large volumes of candidate materials for standard development from recovered patients and blood donors. The main candidate material had now been evaluated in a large number of participating laboratories and was scheduled for lyophilization. An international collaborative study will then evaluate the material using a range of serological and virus neutralization assays. In the case of the HEV reference panel, large volumes of plasma and serum had been collected from Europe and Asia, again from recovered patients and blood donors. Initial characterization of a candidate panel had been performed at PEI and this was currently being evaluated using different enzyme immunoassay formats. All materials were reported to be of high-titre and IgG or IgM positive.

Good progress had also been made in the further expansion of the First WHO International Reference Repository of platelet transfusion-relevant bacterial reference strains. Strains had been selected and manufacturing batches tested for stability. During the period 2017–2018, a total of 17 laboratories worldwide were testing the strains by artificially contaminating red blood cell bags and following bacterial growth kinetics for 42 days. Statistical analysis of the results of these studies was scheduled to start in 2019.

In addition, PEI had taken part in discussions on the importance of demonstrating the commutability of WHO international standards, with agreement reached on the need for additional studies. PEI support was also provided during the development of: (a) the new WHO Recommendations to assure the quality, safety and efficacy of recombinant hepatitis E vaccines (see section 3.4.1); (b) the revised WHO Guidelines for the safe development and production of vaccines to human influenza pandemic viruses and influenza viruses with pandemic potential (see section 3.4.2); and (c) the revised WHO Guidelines for the safe production and quality control of poliomyelitis vaccines (see section 3.4.3). PEI was also involved in the ongoing development of the new WHO Recommendations on RSV vaccines, and in the updating of the WHO Guidelines for assuring the quality and nonclinical evaluation of DNA vaccines.

As in previous years, PEI continued to provide support to the WHO prequalification programme through the reviewing of product files and participation in GMP inspections. PEI involvement in NRA capacity-building activities included support for the self-benchmarking assessments organized by WHO and carried out by NRAs of the Economic Community of West African States. PEI had also been involved in the benchmarking of blood regulatory systems in a number of selected African countries using the WHO GBT blood module. In all cases, support was given to participating countries in identifying their current regulatory strengths and weaknesses, and in developing institutional plans to address identified gaps. Further collaboration with BRN on the development of benchmarking indicators for blood regulatory systems and their integration into the WHO GBT was ongoing.

The Committee thanked Dr Meyer for her report and noted the progress being made with interest.

Center for Biologics Evaluation and Research (CBER), Silver Springs, MD USA

Dr Jay Epstein highlighted a number of recent and current activities at CBER with a specific focus on its participation in WHO collaborative studies to develop and evaluate new international standards and reagents. Examples included the study to develop a WHO international standard for anti-Asian lineage Zika virus antibody (human) and the study to develop a WHO international reference serum for use in RSV-neutralization assays. Considerable support had also been provided in the development of new vaccine technologies. Examples here included the publishing of results from the first collaborative spiking study from the Advanced Virus Detection Interest Group (sponsored by the Parenteral Drug Association) which had evaluated the detection of five distinct viruses using different next-generation sequencing (NGS) platforms, and the continued maintenance of an updated reference virus database to facilitate novel adventitious virus detection by NGS.

Other CBER activities in the vaccine field had included participation in the calibration of influenza reference reagents for seasonal and pandemic influenza viruses. CBER continues to play a crucial role in preparing candidate vaccine viruses (CVVs) for both seasonal and pandemic influenza strains for testing and distribution to WHOCCs and WHO essential regulatory laboratories (ERLs). Studies into alternative methods to the single radial immunodiffusion (SRD) assay for measuring the potency of inactivated influenza vaccines were continuing under the sponsorship of the International Federation of Pharmaceutical Manufacturers & Associations. Recent results had indicated that some mAbs used in alternative potency assays were impacted by the method used to inactivate reference antigen preparations.

CBER had also been centrally involved in a number of projects in the IVD field in recent years. This included the development of the First WHO reference reagents for dengue virus serotypes 1–4 for nucleic acid amplification technique (NAT)-based assays, and the provision and testing of heat-inactivated materials during the development of WHO international standards for chikungunya virus RNA and Zika virus RNA for NAT-based assays. Currently, NIBSC is developing a WHO international standard for West Nile virus RNA for which CBER again provided heat-inactivated virus stock. Dr Epstein also updated the Committee on the current status of work to develop a First WHO International Reference for *Babesia microti* antibodies, a project endorsed by the Committee in 2015. CBER had also developed lot release and reference panels for HIV p24 antigen using primary isolates of HIV-1 subtypes. HIV-1 subtype B and group O lot release panels had been formulated at target concentrations and stored at −70 °C. It was intended that other, non-B subtypes, would also be formulated into an HIV-1 p24 antigen reference panel.

CBER continued to distribute a range of blood products standards and to participate in collaborative studies in this area. Dr Epstein alerted the Committee to the limited remaining supply of the Second WHO International Standard for thrombin. This reference material is used by IVD and haemostasis product manufacturers and it was recommended that consideration be given to the development of a replacement standard. After noting the involvement of CBER in several collaborative studies of blood coagulation factor standards, Dr Epstein further recommended that consideration be given to conducting a collaborative study to establish a first WHO International Standard for activated blood coagulation factor X (FXa) to replace the existing First WHO International Reference Reagent for FXa.

Dr Epstein concluded by reminding the Committee that a wide range of WHO standards development activities are supported by the CBER-WHO Cooperative Agreement process. Examples included the development of modelling approaches to support regulatory decision-making to protect the blood supply from emerging infectious diseases, the revision of the WHO Guidelines for the safe development and production of vaccines to human influenza pandemic viruses and influenza viruses with pandemic potential (see section 3.4.2) and the risk–benefit assessment of the platform technologies used to address priority pathogens defined in the WHO R&D Blueprint.

The Committee thanked Dr Epstein for his report and noted the progress being made with interest.

2.4 Cross-cutting activities of other WHO committees and groups

2.4.1 Update from the WHO Expert Committee on Specifications for Pharmaceutical Preparations

Dr Sabine Kopp updated the Committee on the work of the WHO Expert Committee on Specifications for Pharmaceutical Preparations (ECSPP) which had met in Geneva on 22–26 October 2018. The ECSPP agenda had included several important topics of interest to the Committee, including the content and use of the WHO EML, antimicrobial resistance, ICDRA and the use of international nonproprietary names (INN) for pharmaceutical substances. The Committee was informed that a revised WHO Biowaiver List of products based on the WHO EML had now been approved by the ECSPP. In addition, it had been agreed that, in view of increasing microbial resistance globally, the available chemical standards for antibiotics should be reviewed to see if any action was required.

A number of WHO written standards had been recommended by the ECSPP for adoption, including WHO Guidelines on GMP for heating, ventilation and air-conditioning systems, and WHO Guidelines on GMP for validation – with the latter incorporating: (a) the validation of computerized systems; (b) validation of importation procedures for medicines; (c) validation of quality management systems for NRA GMP inspection; and (d) revised guidance on cleaning validation. In addition, the revision of the European Pharmacopoeia monograph and GMP requirements for water for injection had been discussed at the ECSPP meeting, along with a number of collaborative initiatives on GMP inspection guidelines and good practices between the Pharmaceutical Inspection Co-operation Scheme and WHO and between the ECSPP and the International Atomic Energy Agency on radiopharmaceuticals. Improvements had also been made to the WHO certification scheme on the quality of pharmaceutical products moving in international commerce.

The ECSPP also oversees the revision of the International Pharmacopoeia and the establishment of International Chemical Reference Substances. Dr Kopp reported that eight new chemical entities had been established by the ECSPP as international standards. In addition, the development of a CD Rom and memory stick of the International Pharmacopoeia had now been completed.

The Committee thanked Dr Kopp for her update and noted the developments outlined with interest.

2.4.2 Report of the 67th WHO International Nonproprietary Names Consultation: update on nomenclature for advanced therapies

Dr James Robertson presented an overview of developments in the nomenclature used for advanced therapies – a field which is now rapidly progressing (see section 3.3.1). Dr Robertson used the example of the antiviral "oseltamivir" to explain the INN structure, which consists of a fantasy preface (oselt-) then a substem/inflix (-amivir) for neuraminidase inhibitors which incorporates the stem/suffix for all antivirals (-vir).

INN naming schemes for chemical substances are relatively easy to apply but biologicals have much more complex and heterogeneous structures, and new classes of biotherapeutics require new naming schemes. Considerable difficulties had been encountered in this regard, including in the proposing of new INNs by manufacturers. A code book had now been made available to support the process of nomenclature assignment. The conclusion of the INN consultation was that if the benefits of having an INN outweigh those of not having an INN then an INN should be provided. Stakeholders in this field include prescribers, pharmacists, trademark offices, pharmacopoeias, researchers, regulators and patients, and their views and needs must be taken into account when assessing the likely benefits.

In discussions of INNs for advanced therapies, a recent consultation had considered substances used for cellular and gene therapy and for virus-based therapy. As has always been the case, decisions on the nomenclature used for vaccines are part of the remit of the WHO Expert Committee on Biological Standardization. Dr Robertson proceeded to explain in some detail the naming schemes for substances from the different groups of advanced therapies. Specific issues raised at the consultation and during previous discussions with stakeholders included ongoing concerns about the two-word nomenclature scheme devised for genetically modified autologous cell therapies. In order to support applicants in the construction of an INN and to provide information to health-care professionals on how to interpret an INN, an online "School of INN" had been established. This virtual teaching platform creates online teaching modules, publishes papers and interacts with universities.

The Committee thanked Dr Robertson for his report and for his explanation of the complexities involved in designing and deciphering an INN. The Committee remained of the view that the INN nomenclature proposed for cell therapy products was complicated and likely to be challenging to most of the field, with potential consequences for its use in practice. The Committee looked forward to being updated on the progress made in the nomenclature of advanced therapy products at its future meetings.

2.4.3 Update from the WHO National Control Laboratory Network for Biologicals

Mr Mike Ward reported on the work of the recently formed WHO National Control Laboratory Network for Biologicals (WHO-NNB) in the testing and release of WHO-prequalified vaccines and other prequalified biological products. The main objective of WHO-NNB is to share quality information in order to facilitate access to prequalified vaccines through recognition by

WHO Technical Report Series, No. 1016, 2019

recipient countries of the lot release decision of the responsible NRA. It is intended that this will reduce redundant testing, promote the development of harmonized common standards and facilitate the sharing of best practices.

The first general meeting of this new network had taken place in 2017 at the National Institute of Biologicals, Noida, and had involved more than 20 national control laboratories (NCLs) responsible for the testing of prequalified vaccines, manufacturers' associations and other stakeholders. Participant NCLs were drawn from both vaccine producer and vaccine recipient countries, with 19 having full network membership and a signed confidentiality agreement with WHO. Meeting participants had agreed: (a) to pursue membership agreements with potential additional members; (b) to continue the development of an electronic information-sharing platform; and (c) to perform the first validation of its function – a process now ongoing. Network members had also agreed to distribute laboratory inventories among contributing laboratories, and to approach manufacturers with a view to extending existing information-sharing agreements. A second general meeting was then held in 2018 at the Istituto Superiore di Sanitá, Rome, at which the operations of the network, the sharing of best practices and new developments, and the harmonization of quality control methods had been discussed. A third meeting was planned to take place during 2019 at the South Africa National Control Laboratory for Biological Products, Bloemfontein. Meeting reports are available on the WHO website and in the quarterly journal WHO Drug Information.

The Committee thanked Mr Ward for his report and looked forward to receiving further updates on the work of this important network at its future meetings.

2.4.4 Update from the WHO Product Development for Vaccines Advisory Committee

Dr Birgitte Giersing updated the Committee on the outcomes of the 2018 convening of the WHO Product Development for Vaccines Advisory Committee (PDVAC). Now in its fifth year, PDVAC had been formed to prioritize and accelerate the development of urgently needed vaccines, with a focus on preferred product characteristics and the development of R&D roadmaps. The scope of PDVAC now included vaccines, mAbs and delivery technologies, with a further focus placed on defining and articulating the full public health value of vaccine and mAb technologies. Landscape analysis had been completed for all PDVAC priority pathogens, with roadmaps developed for three of these – namely, malaria, RSV and Group B streptococci. Dr Giersing also provided an overview of the clinical pipeline status of next-generation vaccines for influenza, malaria, tuberculosis and HIV, along with the pipeline status of vaccines against other PDVAC prioritized pathogens.

The Committee was informed that product developers and funders are looking for acceptable routes to accelerate vaccine development using controlled human infection model (CHIM) studies to identify possible correlates of protection and/or as a proxy for field efficacy. PDVAC was frequently asked to provide guidance on clinical trial design and the utility of CHIM studies as a means of accelerating vaccine development. It was considered that such studies had an important role to play in investigating proof of concept leading to a clearer understanding of the pathogenesis of, and immunity to, the challenge organism, and several such studies were currently under way. Although these can inform understanding of the nature of the immune responses a vaccine might need to elicit in order to be protective, it was recognized that any tentative identification of potential immune correlates of protection would require validation in traditional efficacy studies.

The application of CHIM studies to the study of both live and killed candidate Shigella vaccines is of particular current interest, with a view to possibly accelerating vaccine licensure, policy recommendation and uptake. Dr Giersing provided the Committee with an overview of the current status of work in this area. Of particular relevance to the work of the Committee were the current efforts being made to harmonize Shigella O-antigen ELISAs and the development of appropriate reference reagents. The Committee was informed that NIBSC with financial support from the Bill & Melinda Gates Foundation was to conduct a pilot collaborative study across five Shigella vaccine development groups with a focus on assay harmonization. The advice and support of the Committee was being sought with regard to developing appropriate standards in time for the schedules Phase 2/3 studies which could begin in 2021–2022.

The Committee thanked Dr Giersing for her update on the activities of PDVAC and on the status of vaccine development activities globally. Regarding the specific request made for support in the development of appropriate and timely standards for use in Shigella O-antigen assays, the Committee noted that the development of interim standards might provide an immediate way forward. These could subsequently be upgraded to WHO International Standard status once relevant collaborative studies had been carried out and the data found to be satisfactory. The Committee also recognized that awareness of the activities of PDVAC could be very useful when prioritizing the preparation of WHO written standards for new vaccines and the revision of existing ones.

2.4.5 Update on immunization policy from the Strategic Advisory Group of Experts on Immunization

Dr Joachim Hombach reported on the meeting of the Strategic Advisory Group of Experts (SAGE) on Immunization held in October 2018 in Geneva. Meeting topics had included the current state of the Global Vaccine Action Plan, poliomyelitis vaccination, human papillomavirus (HPV) vaccines, use

WHO Technical Report Series, No. 1016, 2019

of measles and rubella vaccines, and Ebola and other unlicensed vaccines for emergency use. Dr Hombach noted that although SAGE recognized the progress being made towards the goals set out in the Global Vaccine Action Plan, it considered that many of the targets were unlikely to be attained by the end of the decade, and that in such a fragile situation there was a risk that hard-won gains could easily be lost. There is therefore still a need to maintain the momentum for immunization efforts and to emphasize its critical importance as a central pillar of UHC. The key role of immunization partners was also highlighted. These include the Global Alliance for Vaccines and Immunization which is undertaking key activities in relation to WHO policy in the areas of typhoid conjugate vaccine, the provision of HPV vaccines to lower-income countries, responding to yellow fever outbreaks and the global stockpile of Ebola vaccine. In addition, the Pregnancy Research Ethics for Vaccines, Epidemics, and New Technologies initiative funded by the Wellcome Trust is committed to developing firm, actionable and consensus-driven ethics guidance on how to equitably include the interests of pregnant women and their offspring (< 5 years old) in the development and deployment of vaccines against emerging pathogens. SAGE welcomed this initiative and during discussions highlighted the need for careful risk–benefit assessments when studying live vaccines in pregnant women.

SAGE had also been presented with a global update on measles and rubella elimination efforts. While noting the substantial progress made in the reduction of global measles incidence and mortality since 2000, SAGE had also expressed its concerns about the loss of the measles elimination status for the WHO Region of the Americas and some countries in the WHO European Region, and the resurgence of measles in four of the six WHO Regions compared to 2016. New data on the co-administration of rubella and measles containing vaccines and yellow fever vaccine had also been presented with SAGE recommending that these vaccines can either be co-administered or administered at least 4 weeks apart. A new guidance document developed to help countries identify and address measles and rubella immunity gaps had now been endorsed by SAGE. However, it was also stressed that as vaccination campaigns are resource intensive and not sustainable, countries should prioritize the strengthening of routine immunization activities.

Dr Hombach reported that SAGE had also welcomed the launch by the Director-General of WHO of the multi-stakeholder "Call For Action: Toward Cervical Cancer Elimination" in May 2018. SAGE considered that the 2017 WHO vaccine position paper remains valid and that a girls-only vaccination programme with coverage of > 80% could lead to the elimination of HPV in most countries and regions without the need for changes to current screening practices. However, major concerns were expressed about the global HPV vaccine supply in the short to mid-term and SAGE urged the globally equitable allocation of available doses, especially to regions with the highest number of cases.

With regard to Ebola and other unlicensed vaccines for emergency use, SAGE had been informed that 13 candidate Ebola vaccines had undergone, or were currently undergoing, clinical trial evaluation. Progress had also been made in the implementation of the expanded access (compassionate use) protocol in the Democratic Republic of the Congo, with > 20 000 at-risk individuals having received the rVSV-ZEBOV vaccine. Modelling studies suggested that ring vaccination would work best in reducing outbreak duration and case numbers if implemented in conjunction with the reactive vaccination of health-care and front-line workers and full implementation of other non-vaccine outbreak control measures. Due to limited data, the risks of administering the live virus vaccine rVSVΔG-ZEBOV-GP to pregnant women remain largely unknown, and decisions on this complex issue would rest with the local NRA and local Ethics Review Committee. SAGE considered the development of non-replicating candidate Ebola vaccines to be a high priority since such vaccines raised fewer safety concerns for use in pregnancy. Supporting NRAs in Ebola endemic countries in the development of regulatory pathways leading to the evaluation and licensure of candidate Ebola vaccines also remained an urgent priority.

The Committee thanked Dr Hombach for his update and noted the availability of the full SAGE meeting report in the WHO *Weekly Epidemiological Record* (https://apps.who.int/iris/bitstream/handle/10665/276544/WER9349. pdf?ua=1). It was noted that ring vaccination does not always go well due to population movement and other local concerns such as access and security. Mention was also made of the potential role of the WHO EUAL procedure in compassionate use situations. Agreement was expressed for the clear need to assess candidate Ebola vaccines other than rVSVΔG-ZEBOV-GP for clinical end-points. The WHO Guidelines on the quality, safety and efficacy of Ebola vaccines adopted at the 2017 meeting of the Committee were available along with WHO international reference preparations for Ebola antibodies and Ebola RNA, but there is some uncertainty concerning the degree to which these resources were currently being used.

2.4.6 Progress report on the WHO pilot procedure for the prequalification of biotherapeutic products and SBPs

Dr Deus Mubangizi reported on the progress of a WHO pilot procedure for the prequalification of biotherapeutic products or their corresponding SBPs which is specifically focused on rituximab and trastuzumab. The pilot procedure will be carried out using either full or abridged assessment pathways. The full assessment pathway would be applied to SBPs that have been registered by non-stringent regulatory authorities using an SRA-approved reference biological product as comparator, and that are marketed in the authorized country. An abridged assessment pathway would be used when innovator products or SBPs for rituximab and trastuzumab have been approved for marketing by an SRA.

WHO Technical Report Series, No. 1016, 2019

The pilot procedure had been introduced in a concept note in May 2017 and, following public consultation, guidelines had been finalized in June 2018. A public call for expressions of interest in making a submission had been issued in July 2018. In accordance with the risk-based assessment approach to be used, the assessment of an SRA-approved product will primarily involve independent "verification" focusing on labelling, storage and identicality. For non-SRA-approved products, a full assessment will be made by WHO, with the possibility of independent laboratory testing and inspections. The WHO prequalification assessment process will include assistance from external experts in biotherapeutic products and SBPs.

Dr Mubangizi explained that the purpose of WHO prequalification of rituximab and trastuzumab and of their associated SBPs was to provide United Nations agencies, international, regional and national procurement agencies, and WHO Member States with guidance on the acceptability of candidate products that meet WHO technical guidance on quality, safety and efficacy or performance. This will include compliance with good laboratory practice, GMP, good clinical practice and good distribution practice, and the meeting of relevant operational packaging and presentation specifications. By submitting an expression of interest, an applicant undertakes to share information with WHO on all relevant aspects of manufacture and control of the specified products and on any changes made and/or planned. Applicants are also expected to provide a risk management plan and to promptly communicate to WHO any safety concerns relating to the products.

Successful completion of the prequalification procedure will result in a Letter of prequalification to the applicant, and publication on the WHO website of the WHO list of prequalified products, and associated public assessment and public inspection reports. Maintenance of the WHO list of prequalified products will involve sampling and testing, handling of variations and complaints, re-inspection and re-qualification, as appropriate. WHO may suspend or remove products from the list and negative evaluation outcomes will also be published, including notices of concern and suspension as applicable. Dr Mubangizi emphasized that WHO prequalified products must still be approved for use by NRAs as WHO prequalification does not substitute for NRA market approval. A list of frequently asked questions relating to the pilot procedure had also been prepared. To date, WHO had received one formal application, with interest having been expressed by other manufacturers in a number of countries. A list of assessors and GMP inspectors had been drawn up. It is intended that various aspects of the pilot procedure will be evaluated one year after its launch in July 2019.

The Committee thanked Dr Mubangizi for his report and raised several points for consideration by the WHO Prequalification Team in relation to the selection of testing laboratories, the specific aspects to be tested, and the appropriateness of the risk-management plans in low- and middle-income countries (LMIC) for monitoring SBPs. The Committee looked forward with interest to being updated in due course on the progress made by this initiative.

2.4.7 WHO Global model regulatory framework for medical devices including in vitro diagnostic medical devices

Dr Adriana Velazquez outlined to the Committee the key role of medical devices, including IVDs, in achieving the Sustainable Development Goal 3: Ensure healthy lives and promote well-being for all at all ages. Medical devices are health technologies that include IVDs, implantable devices, surgical instruments, and medical equipment and software. Ensuring access to good quality and safe medical devices following innovation and product development requires appropriate regulatory oversight, including assessment of safety and clinical effectiveness, as well as the management of procurement and use. The Committee was informed that there have been two World Health Assembly resolutions on strengthening national regulatory systems, in particular systems which are the least developed such as those for medical devices including IVDs. To facilitate improved access to, and use of, quality medical devices, the WHO *Global model regulatory framework for medical devices including in vitro diagnostic medical devices* had now been developed. The framework sets out guiding principles and harmonized definitions, and specifies the attributes of effective and efficient regulation to be embodied within binding and enforceable law. While additional benefits may be expected to accrue from the WHO model regulatory framework, its primary objectives are to provide a robust framework to promote trust and confidence in medical devices, enable efficient use of regulatory resources and encourage continuous improvement in regulatory systems.

Dr Velazquez then outlined the objectives of the recently developed WHO Model List of Essential In Vitro Diagnostics (EDL) which lists IVDs recommended by WHO for use at various levels of a tiered laboratory system. The EDL is expected to provide guidance to Member States on the development of local essential diagnostics lists and to inform United Nations agencies and nongovernmental organizations working in the selection, procurement, supply, donation or provision of IVDs. The EDL will also provide guidance to the medical technology private sector on diagnostics priorities for addressing global health issues. The first edition of the EDL (2018) covers a range of tests for "high-priority" infectious diseases plus general laboratory tests, but no brand names or specific products. An annual review of the EDL will be conducted under the oversight of the newly established Strategic Advisory Group of Experts on In Vitro Diagnostics (see section 2.4.8) using a process similar to that currently used for the WHO EML. The inclusion of IVDs in the list will be based on public health relevance, and will be evidence based and free of conflict of interests. For each test listed, a link will be provided to any WHO-prequalified products if available, as well as any to relevant WHO supporting documents. A dedicated WHO web portal was in the process of being established to bring together all WHO information resources relevant to IVDs in order to support laboratory capacity development in WHO Member States. Dr Velazquez then outlined a number of anticipated future needs in areas such as the building up of regulatory support in countries for IVD market approval, the development of technical specifications for IVD procurement and laboratory capacity-building in the IVD sector. Dr Velazquez concluded by highlighting the upcoming 4th Global Forum on Medical Devices to be held in Visakhapatnam in December 2018.

The Committee thanked Dr Velazquez for her presentation and noted the considerable developments that had taken place in WHO activities to promote access to and use of medical devices, including IVDs. There would be a need for the Committee to work closely with the newly established Strategic Advisory Group of Experts on In Vitro Diagnostics to identify priorities in this area.

2.4.8 First meeting of the Strategic Advisory Group of Experts on In Vitro Diagnostics

Dr Clare Morris informed the Committee that the Strategic Advisory Group of Experts on In Vitro Diagnostics (SAGE IVD) had held its first meeting in April 2018. The meeting had consisted of four days of closed meetings together with a one-day open session with external stakeholders. The 19 invited members of SAGE IVD were drawn from 15 countries and included programme directors, technical directors and professors working in a variety of specialties covering both infectious and noncommunicable diseases. Additional advisors from a range of WHO programme areas had also attended specific sessions of the meeting, with Professor Klaus Cichutek, Dr Lery, Dr Knezevic and Dr Morris attending as observers on behalf of the Committee.

Previously, some initial concerns had been expressed regarding the potential for overlap between the role of SAGE IVD and the activities of the Committee. However, SAGE IVD is tasked with the development of the WHO EDL – akin to the WHO EML – and issues of standardization were not addressed during discussions. An overview of the Committee and its role, with examples of the importance of standardization in diagnostics, had been presented at the meeting. SAGE IVD emphasized the need to work collaboratively and expressed the view that there was no need for SAGE IVD to cover work already addressed by other WHO entities. It was indicated that the Committee would be happy to provide updates on its work in this area at future SAGE IVD meetings to promote complementary working arrangements.

SAGE IVD had agreed that the development of an EDL would support strategic WHO priorities such as UHC, help to address health emergencies and promote healthier populations. It was also agreed that priority should be given to IVDs needed for progress towards UHC with a focus on tests relevant to WHO priority diseases – HIV, tuberculosis, malaria, viral hepatitis, syphilis and HPV. A process for editing the EDL was agreed and an annual update would be expected. Priority in the first round of revisions would be given to antimicrobial resistance, neglected tropical diseases, PHEs and sepsis.

It was considered that the WHO EDL and WHO prequalification of IVDs were complementary processes in improving access to IVDs for Member States. However, following a number of clarifications regarding the processes to be followed for the approval of prequalification documents and selection of IVDs for prequalification review, SAGE IVD considered that WHO prequalification was neither necessary nor sufficient for the inclusion of an IVD in the EDL.

It was expected that the EDL would be expanded in the coming years, in line with the WHO priority of progressing towards the goals of UHC. SAGE IVD membership would be partially refreshed annually but the recruitment mechanism for new members was not yet clear.

The Committee thanked Dr Morris for her report and looked forward to seeing the published SAGE IVD meeting report in due course. The Committee agreed on the importance of working closely with SAGE IVD in order to maximize progress in the priority areas noted, and highlighted the need to further explore the best ways of achieving this.

3. International Recommendations, Guidelines and other matters related to the manufacture, quality control and evaluation of biological substances

3.1 General

3.1.1 Revision of the WHO Recommendations for the preparation, characterization and establishment of international and other biological reference standards[7]

The Committee was reminded that a proposal to update the above WHO Recommendations had been discussed at its meeting in 2017. Following highly detailed and wide-ranging technical discussion, it had been concluded that revision and updating of the current guidance was evidently needed given the numerous issues previously raised. It had further recommended that any revision process should take into consideration the needs of different target audiences by seeking their views and inputs. Indeed, it had been suggested that consideration might usefully be given to exploring the need for a companion document directed primarily towards end users of WHO international standards and other reference preparations which could include guidance on the calibration of secondary standards, as well as broader metrological considerations. The Committee had requested that the broad range of issues raised be discussed by WHOCCs and that specific proposals be presented to the Committee for consideration at its next meeting. The Committee was informed that such discussions had now taken place during 2018.

At its meeting in April 2018, the WHO network of collaborating centres for blood products and in vitro diagnostics had agreed that the current document would benefit from updating, particularly given its insufficient coverage of the diagnostics field. During discussion, a request was made for a gap analysis of the document to be conducted to determine whether a simple update to include diagnostics or a complete rewrite of the whole document was required. The analysis had duly been completed and a wide range of issues identified. These included the need for a clearer overall document structure, improved definitions of key concepts, improved clarity in areas such as unit assignment and commutability, and the updating of examples and possible replacement of the current appendix.

---

[7] Recommendations for the preparation, characterization and establishment of international and other biological reference standards. In: WHO Expert Committee on Biological Standardization: fifty-fifth report. Geneva: World Health Organization; 2005: Annex 2 (WHO Technical Report Series, No. 932; https://apps.who.int/iris/bitstream/handle/10665/43278/WHO_TRS_932_eng.pdf?sequence=1, accessed 9 March 2019).

The same gap analysis was subsequently presented to the WHO network of collaborating centres on standardization and regulatory evaluation of vaccines at its meeting in September 2018 (see section 2.2.2). It was recognized that the current document was intended for use by WHOCCs and that an update would be beneficial. Discussions centred on how pressing such an update was, and on whether or not a revised document needed to have WHO Recommendations status and be published in the official report of the Committee. It was suggested that a document that would only be available to WHOCCs would allow for greater flexibility in terms of its future updating. The network considered that developing a separate document outlining the use of international reference preparations for end users was a more pressing need. Such a document could be used to support the uptake and adoption of the use of IU which would benefit patient health care through improved global standardization. As the needs of vaccine, diagnostic and biotherapeutic end users are different, the question of producing several appropriately tailored documents was also raised.

In summary, the overall conclusion of these consultations had been that the revision of the current WHO Recommendations was needed but not essential. However, end user guidance was urgently required. It had been proposed that a dedicated workshop on this subject should first be held to help shape the creation of any new guidance document(s) and to inform appropriate revision. Consideration would need to be given to how such a workshop could be funded and hosted, and to the ways in which other related planned workshops could be utilized.

The Committee expressed its thanks for the clear and comprehensive assessment provided of the need to update the WHO Recommendations for the preparation, characterization and establishment of international and other biological reference standards. Following discussion and clarification of various points, the Committee recommended that WHO should first consider holding a workshop to explore further the nature and content of any new document(s), focusing first on an end users document and bearing in mind the already available WHO Manual for the preparation of secondary reference materials for in vitro diagnostic assays designed for infectious disease nucleic acid or antigen detection: calibration to WHO International Standards.

3.1.2   WHO Vero reference cell bank 10-87

The WHO Vero reference cell bank (RCB) 10-87 was originally established in 1987 and is a unique resource for the development of biological medicines for which a cell substrate with a safe and reliable history is needed. WHO Vero RCB 10-87 is considered to be suitable for use as a cell seed for generating a master cell bank (MCB) and is stored at the European Collection of Animal Cell

Cultures in the United Kingdom and at the American Type Culture Collection in the USA. In 2002, following expert review, its name was changed from "WHO Vero cell bank 10-87" to "WHO Vero reference cell bank 10-87" to better reflect its status as a cell seed suitable for generating an MCB rather than a cell bank in its own right.

The Committee was informed that only a limited number of vials now remained with their distribution now restricted solely to the production of vaccines and other biologicals. The development of a replacement RCB had previously been discussed without resolution, and would be an expensive and time consuming process involving the preparation, testing and maintenance of the new RCB. It was also unclear whether the preparation of a new RCB should be carried out under full GMP or under GMP-like conditions.

An increasing number of requests for the WHO Vero RCB 10-87 were now being received from Chinese manufacturers and the question had arisen of whether NIFDC could establish a national Vero cell bank. NIFDC had requested clarification of whether such a material should be prepared and stored under full GMP or in a GMP-like facility. This same issue had been discussed at the 2018 meeting of the WHO network of collaborating centres on standardization and regulatory evaluation of vaccines held in Beijing and similar clarification sought.

Following consideration, the Committee concluded that a replacement WHO Vero RCB 10-87 could be produced under GMP-like conditions rather than full GMP. There was general consensus that the most important point to emphasize is that the WHO Vero RCB 10-87 – like the WHO RCB of MRC-5 cells (see section 9.1.1) – is not considered suitable for direct use as an MCB for the production of licensed products but rather as a defined and well-characterized cell seed with a detailed history and database. With its excellent traceability to the original cells and to the materials used in the preparation of the seed stock, the WHO Vero RCB 10-87 is provided to manufacturers in order to generate an MCB for use in production. The MCB would of course need to be produced and tested under full GMP according to current WHO Recommendations,[8] which clearly state that "GMP should be applied from the stage of cell banking onwards" and that cell lines "should originate from well-characterized and qualified sources and the cells from an appropriately qualified seed stock or MCB".

---

[8] Recommendations for the evaluation of animal cell cultures as substrates for the manufacture of biological medicinal products and for the characterization of cell banks. In: WHO Expert Committee on Biological Standardization: sixty-first report. Geneva: World Health Organization; 2013: Annex 3 (WHO Technical Report Series, No. 978; http://www.who.int/biologicals/vaccines/TRS_978_Annex_3.pdf, accessed 14 March 2019).

3.1.3 Deletion of the innocuity/abnormal toxicity test for biological products

The Committee was reminded that the innocuity test (also referred to as the abnormal toxicity test or general safety test) is a quality control test carried out on the final product for the purpose of licensing or lot release. Developed in the early 1900s, the test was intended to ensure the safe and consistent production of serum products and later became a general safety test to detect extraneous contaminants in all biological products. The test has historically been included in WHO Recommendations and Guidelines from the onset and in national pharmacopoeias worldwide.

In recent years, however, the value of the test has been called into question – both from the perspective of regulatory science and in the context of the principles of animal use. The Committee was reminded that one of the main outcomes of a 2015 conference of the International Alliance for Biological Standardization on the 3Rs concept was a formal request to WHO to initiate steps to delete the innocuity test from all WHO Recommendations, Guidelines and other WHO written standards. A number of international initiatives had already been taken in this direction, including revocation of the general safety test regulations in 2015 by the US FDA, which considered them no longer necessary or appropriate in helping to ensure the safety, purity and potency of licensed biological products. In addition, in 2017, the European Pharmacopoeia Commission endorsed the complete suppression of the innocuity test from the European Pharmacopoeia with effect from 1 January 2019. The position of WHO had also changed in recent years. Prior to 2000, the test was required on each final lot with subsequent guidance indicating that the test could be omitted during routine lot release once consistency of production had been established. The position of WHO changed again in 2015 when the Committee advised that the need to test final vaccine lots for unexpected toxicity using the innocuity test should be agreed with the NRA. It was further noted in small print that some countries no longer required this test.

The scientific rationale and evidence for performing the innocuity test as a measure of the safety of vaccines and other biological products for the purpose of marketing authorization and lot release were discussed in depth by the Committee. Current manufacturing processes, which include the implementation of GMP and comprehensive quality control measures (including in-process controls), were considered to be more appropriate than the innocuity test in assuring the quality and safety of vaccines and other biological products. The Committee then reviewed the historical inclusion of the innocuity test in documents published in the WHO Technical Report Series and concluded that its complete omission would not compromise the quality and safety of vaccines and other biological products. As a result, the Committee recommended the immediate discontinuation of the inclusion of the innocuity test in all future WHO Recommendations, Guidelines and manuals for biological products published in the Technical Report Series. The Committee further recommended that the inclusion of this test in previously published WHO Technical Report Series documents be disregarded. It was considered that these recommendations represented a significant step towards science-based regulation and regulatory convergence at the global level.

3.2 Biotherapeutics other than blood products

3.2.1 WHO Questions and Answers: similar biotherapeutic products

The WHO Guidelines on evaluation of similar biotherapeutic products (SBPs) were adopted in 2009 and have raised global awareness of the complex scientific issues involved in the licensing of SBPs. In May 2014, the Sixty-seventh World Health Assembly adopted a new resolution on improving access to biotherapeutic products, including SBPs, and ensuring their quality, safety and efficacy. One of the requests made in the resolution was for the Committee to "update the 2009 guidelines, taking into account the technological advances for the characterization of biotherapeutic products and considering national regulatory needs and capacities". In response, WHO convened a series of meetings, including a WHO informal consultation in 2015 during which it was agreed that the evaluation principles described in the 2009 Guidelines were still valid, valuable and applicable in facilitating the harmonization of SBP regulatory requirements globally. It was however concluded that there was a need for additional guidance on the evaluation of mAb products as SBPs. Such guidance was subsequently developed, recommended by the Committee for adoption and published in 2017.[9]

In May 2017, WHO held another consultation on improving access to and use of SBPs, following which it was agreed that a WHO questions-and-answers document to be read in conjunction with the 2009 Guidelines would be an appropriate way of further clarifying and complementing some of the issues and points covered in the Guidelines. A draft document had therefore been prepared based on the questions most frequently asked by regulators during the Guideline implementation workshops held in the past nine years. The draft document WHO/BS/2018.2352 had then been subjected to two rounds of public consultation and comments received on how to improve its content and

[9] Guidelines on evaluation of monoclonal antibodies as similar biotherapeutic products (SBPs). In: WHO Expert Committee on Biological Standardization: sixty-seventh report. Geneva: World Health Organization; 2017: Annex 2 (WHO Technical Report Series, No. 1004; http://who.int/biologicals/biotherapeutics/WHO_TRS_1004_web_Annex_2.pdf?ua=1, accessed 15 March 2019).

clarity. It was emphasized to the Committee that the resulting document was intended for guidance only and was to be read in conjunction with the relevant WHO guidelines.

Following considerable discussion and several further amendments to the text, the Committee concluded that the WHO Question and Answers: similar biotherapeutic products document (WHO/BS/2018.2352) would be a suitable and helpful resource for supporting the interpretation of the 2009 WHO Guidelines. The Committee recommended that it be adopted and posted on the WHO website rather than published as an annex to its report. The Committee asked that any future updates to the document be brought to its attention. The Committee recognized that the 2009 WHO Guidelines remained valid and did not therefore require revision at this point. Instead the complementary questions-and-answers document should be read and interpreted in conjunction with the two WHO Guidelines on the evaluation of SBPs and of mAbs used as SBPs. Taken together, these three documents would provide up-to-date guidance on the evaluation of SBPs.

3.3 Cellular and gene therapies

3.3.1 Update on cellular and gene therapies

The Committee was updated on developments and progress in this highly active area that had taken place since its previous meeting. The Committee was first reminded that in May 2014 the Sixty-seventh World Health Assembly had adopted resolution WHA67.20 to "increase support and guidance for strengthening the capacity to regulate increasingly complex biological products ... and, where appropriate ... somatic-cell therapy". At its 2017 meeting, the Committee had recommended that WHO collaborate with other international groups active in the area of cellular and gene therapies in developing a common guideline document. Although a variety of relevant guidelines and regulations currently exist or are in development by both governmental and professional organizations in different regions of the world, there is a need to identify common principles for the regulatory evaluation of these products. The harmonizing of definitions and terminology would be particularly helpful for countries that are in the processes of setting out their own national requirements. Clarification of whether genetically modified cells should be included or considered under gene therapy should be provided, and such guidance should include both somatic cell and stem cell therapies.

This issue had also been discussed at the 2018 ICDRA at which a recommendation had been made that WHO develop in collaboration with its Member States a state-of-the-art document capturing areas where agreement among experienced regulatory authorities exists, noting where harmonization has yet to be achieved, and documenting areas of uncertainty. ICDRA had also

WHO Technical Report Series, No. 1016, 2019

encouraged WHO Member States to develop national guidance and legislation in this area.

Advanced therapy products present a broad range of regulatory challenges with a clear need for the development and strengthening of expertise in the regulatory review of such products in many jurisdictions. In addition, the transition from pilot-scale to commercial manufacturing could be challenging for developers of both cellular and gene therapies and novel approaches to their clinical development were needed due to often limited patient populations for clinical trials. WHO had been active in identifying the many opportunities for collaboration towards regulatory convergence, including collaboration with international groups and initiatives. For example, jointly organized conferences with the International Alliance for Biological Standardization had resulted in a number of publications on the scientific considerations and potential common principles for the regulatory oversight of these novel products. The most recent such initiative in which WHO was involved had been a meeting on the manufacturing and testing of pluripotent stem cells held in Los Angeles in June 2018. The meeting had concluded that there were many opportunities for regulatory convergence, starting with a gap analysis of existing guidelines to determine which issues were not covered and which might be creating divergence. Meeting participants also noted that more specific global regulatory guidance would be welcome, preferably issued by WHO.

The Committee discussed the best way forward and agreed that the standardization of cellular and gene therapies should be included in the work of WHO as an area of great importance from the global public health perspective. The Committee noted the above ICDRA recommendation that WHO develop a state-of-the-art document and encouraged WHO to assign appropriate resources to the setting up of a Working Group on the standardization of cellular and gene therapies to take this work forward. The Committee also agreed that clarification of the terminology used in the regulation of these products would be very helpful.

3.4 Vaccines and related substances

3.4.1 Recommendations to assure the quality, safety and efficacy of recombinant hepatitis E vaccines

HEV is a major cause of sporadic and epidemic hepatitis and is found worldwide. The highest seroprevalence rates are observed in regions with low standards of sanitation. In 2015, the WHO SAGE on Immunization had issued a position paper which reviewed evidence on the burden of hepatitis E and on the safety, immunogenicity, efficacy and cost-effectiveness of a hepatitis E vaccine that was first licensed in China. The WHO Global Advisory Committee on Vaccine Safety had reviewed this same hepatitis E vaccine in 2014 and concluded that it had an acceptable safety profile. In 2016, WHO published its *Global health sector strategy on viral hepatitis 2016–2021*, which addresses hepatitis A, B, C and E – with hepatitis E probably being the most neglected of the four. This strategy document highlighted the urgent need to address all viral hepatitis, including hepatitis E for which only one vaccine is approved anywhere in the world and for which no effective therapies exist.

Although many experimental hepatitis E vaccines have been evaluated in virus challenge studies in non-human primates, other animal models or clinical trials, only one vaccine has been licensed for human use as of mid-2018. This vaccine, based on the capsid protein, was licensed in China in December 2011 for use in persons aged 16 years and over. The Committee was informed that other vaccines based on the HEV capsid protein were currently in nonclinical or clinical development.

Following requests from manufacturers and other stakeholders for WHO guidance in this area, a series of meetings had been convened to review the current status of development and likely time to licensure of such vaccines. A first draft of the WHO Recommendations to assure the quality, safety and efficacy of recombinant hepatitis E vaccines had then been developed taking into consideration the discussions of a WHO working group meeting in Geneva, 11–12 May 2017. Following a round of public consultation and further discussions at a meeting in Beijing, 18–19 April 2018, a second draft document was developed. After a second round of public consultation the current document WHO/BS/2018.2348 had been produced.

The Committee was informed that these WHO Recommendations are intended to provide guidance to NRAs and manufacturers on the manufacturing processes, and nonclinical and clinical evaluations, needed to assure the quality, safety and efficacy of recombinant hepatitis E vaccines. The document encompasses recombinant hepatitis E vaccines for prophylactic use based on the ORF2 capsid protein, and should be read in conjunction with other relevant WHO guidance, especially on the nonclinical and clinical evaluation of vaccines. The Committee was reminded that a WHO reference preparation for HEV antibodies was available for the standardization of diagnostic tests for use in seroprevalence studies and for assessing immunity. WHO international reference preparations for HEV RNA were also available for the calibration of in-house or working standards used in the amplification and detection of HEV RNA.

During discussion, the Committee noted that the document focused on monovalent vaccines based on expression systems in *Escherichia coli*, as is the case for the currently licensed vaccine in China. Based on cross-protection data between HEV genotypes 1–4, there would appear to be no need at present for multivalent vaccines. However, given the lack of evidence for cross-protection against other HEV genotypes (5–7) the Committee recommended that the further development of hepatitis E vaccines should be monitored and the recommendations updated as appropriate in line with vaccine developments.

The Committee also reviewed the main comments received during the development of the document and after making a number of changes to the text, recommended that the document WHO/BS/2018.2348 be adopted and annexed to its report (Annex 2). Following the recommendation of the Committee to henceforth discontinue the inclusion of the innocuity test in all WHO written standards appearing in the Technical Report Series (see section 3.1.3) the WHO Recommendations to assure the quality, safety and efficacy of recombinant hepatitis E vaccines became the first such WHO written standard in which the test does not appear.

3.4.2 Guidelines for the safe development and production of vaccines to human pandemic influenza viruses and influenza viruses with pandemic potential

Careful risk assessment and strict biosafety and biosecurity precautions are needed in laboratory and manufacturing environments in order to ensure the safe handling of human pandemic influenza viruses, CVVs and influenza viruses with pandemic potential (IVPP) as the uncontrolled release of such viruses could have a significant impact on public health. In 2007, the WHO biosafety risk assessment and guidelines for the production and quality control of human influenza pandemic vaccines were published in response to the pandemic threat posed by highly pathogenic avian influenza (HPAI) A(H5N1) viruses and the need to begin vaccine development.

Since then, experience in the use of both IVPP and pandemic influenza viruses in the development and production of CVVs has increased globally. This experience includes the development and testing of CVVs derived by reverse genetics from HPAI viruses. Moreover, in response to the 2009 pandemic caused by the A(H1N1)pdm09 subtype virus and the emergence of low pathogenic avian influenza A(H7N9) viruses that are able to infect humans and cause severe disease with a high case fatality rate, piecemeal updates to the 2007 guidance were produced by WHO and posted on its website. In addition, several WHO consultations on influenza vaccines identified the testing timelines for CVVs as one of the bottlenecks to rapid vaccine responses. In light of these and other developments, requests were made to WHO by industry, regulators and laboratories of the WHO Global Influenza Surveillance and Response System (GISRS) to undertake a complete revision of the 2007 guidance.

In response, WHO convened a working group meeting on 9–10 May 2017 attended by representatives of WHOCCs, ERLs, NRAs for vaccine and biosafety regulation, manufacturers and the World Organisation for Animal Health. The working group reviewed cumulative experience, discussed the revision of the 2007 WHO Guidelines and reached a consensus on the outline and key elements of the revision. A first draft document was then prepared and posted on the WHO website for public consultation. A WHO informal consultation was then held on 23–24 April 2018 to finalize the revision process resulting in the document WHO/BS/2018.2349 which follows the risk assessment scheme used in the WHO biosafety guidance for pilot-lot vaccine production. It also includes considerations relating to the greater scale of production needed to rapidly supply large quantities of vaccines, for which the risks are likely to be different to those for pilot lots. The document also takes into account the considerable experience gained from handling HPAI viruses and those classified as low virulence for avian species but highly virulent for humans.

The Committee was informed that the revised WHO Guidelines provide guidance to CVV-testing laboratories, vaccine manufacturers and NRAs on the safe development and production of human influenza vaccines in response to the threat of a pandemic. Updated biosafety expectations for pilot-scale and large-scale vaccine production and laboratory research are also described. The document also specifies the measures to be taken to prevent or minimize the risk to workers involved in the development and production processes, and to prevent or minimize the risk of release of virus into the environment, including the risk of transmission to animals. Tests required to evaluate the safety of CVVs are also described. The document is intended to be read in conjunction with the WHO *Laboratory biosafety manual.*

The Committee noted that the proposed revised Guidelines had undergone further international consultation which had resulted in only a few additional amendments. It also noted that the document takes a conservative but flexible approach. Most of the comments received during public consultation had been related to the safety testing of CVVs. One specific suggestion raised during discussion was that the testing of CVVs in ferrets may not be necessary but this was not accepted given insufficient justification at this time, and given that the Guidelines already allowed for the relaxation of such testing under certain circumstances. For CVVs developed from newly emerging IVPP, a WHO expert group will review the data obtained from safety testing and advise WHO. WHO will then provide further guidance on appropriate containment requirements through its expert networks such as GISRS.

Following a number of further clarifications the Committee recommended that the document WHO/BS/2018.2349 be adopted and annexed to its report (Annex 3).

3.4.3 Guidelines for the safe production and quality control of poliomyelitis vaccines

The Committee was reminded that the WHO Guidelines for the safe production and quality control of inactivated poliomyelitis vaccine manufactured from wild polioviruses had been published in 2004 as an addendum to the previous Recommendations for the production and control of poliomyelitis vaccine (inactivated). These 2004 Guidelines specify the measures to be taken to minimize the risk of accidental reintroduction of wild-type poliovirus from a vaccine manufacturing facility into the community after global certification of polio eradication.

In response to subsequent developments in manufacture and the progress of the polio eradication programme, revised WHO Recommendations for the production of both IPV and oral poliomyelitis vaccine (OPV) had recently also been published. Both of these documents highlight the need for enhanced biorisk management in the production and control of poliomyelitis vaccines after eradication but do not provide detailed guidance on this aspect. Although current guidance emphasizes the need for poliomyelitis vaccine production to comply with GMP and with the containment requirements outlined in the third revision of the WHO Global Action Plan to minimize poliovirus facility-associated risk after type-specific eradication of wild polioviruses and sequential cessation of oral polio vaccine use (GAPIII), none of the currently available guidelines and recommendations provides sufficient detail concerning strategies or approaches for achieving this.

The Committee was informed that the proposed revised WHO Guidelines specifically address the containment measures needed during the production and quality control of IPV produced both from wild-type poliovirus strains and from the live-attenuated vaccine (Sabin) strains used in the manufacture of OPV. They also address the containment measures needed during the production of OPV and IPV produced from novel safer poliovirus strains developed by genetic manipulation. The Committee was informed that the WHO Containment Advisory Group had recently exempted certain of these strains (such as S19) from GAPIII containment requirements for vaccine manufacture and quality control testing. Although the production of poliomyelitis vaccines using platforms involving genetic expression systems without virus replication was outside the scope of the proposed Guidelines, it was expected that any quality control test using live poliovirus should be carried out in a containment facility following the guidance provided by GAPIII and these Guidelines.

As expected, the proposed Guidelines had undergone considerable international review and public consultation, including discussion at three working group meetings. Following the third working group meeting held in Geneva, 7–8 May 2018, the document WHO/BS/2018.2350 had been prepared taking into account all the inputs received. This document had then been subjected to a closing round of public consultation, and the comments and suggestions received were being presented to the Committee for its consideration. It was emphasized that the proposed WHO Guidelines were intended to be read in conjunction with the GAPIII document and with the reports of the WHO Containment Advisory Group.

The Committee reviewed the proposed Guidelines and reflected upon the points raised in the final public consultation. Following discussion and clarification of certain points, the Committee recommended that the document WHO/BS/2018.2350 be adopted and attached to its report (Annex 4). In 2016, the Committee had discussed the importance of these revised Guidelines in the context of GAPIII and of the WHO *Polio Eradication & Endgame Strategic Plan 2013–2018*. It therefore recommended that consideration be given to the holding of implementation workshops to ensure that NRAs, poliomyelitis vaccine manufacturers, researchers and public health officials were aware of and understood the updated guidance provided.

3.4.4 Revision of the WHO Recommendations to assure the quality, safety and efficacy of poliomyelitis vaccines (inactivated)

The Committee was reminded that the above WHO Recommendations had been published in 2015 and had been based on the status of GAPIII during the Guideline development process. At that time, experience with Sabin IPV (sIPV) was limited with only one vaccine of this type having been licensed. Today, many manufacturers were developing sIPV. In addition, GAPIII had since been updated and implemented, thus restricting global laboratory capacity for dealing with wild-type polioviruses. This has now led to difficulties in complying with the requirements of the WHO Recommendations, and requests for urgent clarification of the following issues had been sought, including from several sIPV manufacturers: (a) the recommended tests to be used for confirmation of attenuated vaccine strain phenotype; (b) the testing required to demonstrate effective inactivation, and the cell substrates recommended for use in detecting residual live poliovirus; and (c) the evaluation of immunogenicity in nonclinical and clinical studies.

The Committee was presented with an overview of the major challenges and developments in these three areas. Ensuring the attenuated phenotype of poliovirus seeds and of the purified monovalent virus pool is crucially important as vaccine manufacturing facilities handling attenuated poliovirus are considered to pose a lower biosafety risk than those handling wild-type strains. However, the Committee was informed that due to the implementation of GAPIII measures there was now only limited capacity globally to conduct the in vivo neurovirulence control test recommended in the current WHO Recommendations. It was felt that the more sensitive and validated molecular analysis of nucleotide composition could now be recommended for use in inferring the attenuated phenotype and consistency of the virus seeds and monovalent virus pools used in production. Significant progress had also been made in the selection of cell lines used to test for the effective inactivation of poliovirus. A recent study had shown that the currently recommended primary monkey kidney cells could safely be replaced by the more sensitive continuous cell line L20B. Discussions had also taken place on how best to evaluate IPV immunogenicity in nonclinical and clinical studies and to ensure that any new sIPV provided adequate clinical protection. It was felt that the current requirement for clinical data demonstrating protective neutralizing antibody titres against heterologous poliovirus strain(s) should be retained but that it would be acceptable for such evidence to be generated in a subset of clinical samples. Additionally, this requirement could be waived for tech-transfer products if certain conditions were met. Other strategies may also be acceptable, provided that the data and analysis demonstrate or infer protective immunity against heterologous poliovirus strains. Work was ongoing with a number of WHO programmes to review additional data and evidence, and to evaluate potential alternative approaches to this issue. In conclusion, the Committee was reminded of the urgent need to clarify the situation regarding the status of the current WHO Recommendations. The clinical development of many sIPV products was now under way and both developers and NRAs urgently required guidance in this area.

The Committee thanked the presenters for drawing its attention to the issues raised. Following considerable discussion it was agreed that the WHO Recommendations to assure the quality, safety and efficacy of poliomyelitis vaccines (inactivated) should be updated but that updating the whole document would inevitably take time. Recognizing the urgency of the situation, it was suggested that a public consultation be organized to discuss the three issues raised and that an interim addendum to the WHO Recommendations be developed. However, it was thought that a full public consultation would take some months to organize, as would the potential adoption of an interim addendum. It was proposed that a face-to-face meeting be organized with experts and the Committee to agree on interim measures to deal with the most pressing issues, such as the acceptability of generating neutralization antibody data on only a subset of clinical samples in demonstrating non-inferiority. Whichever pathway was chosen by WHO for moving forward, the Committee indicated its willingness to expedite its decision-making processes so that the outcomes could be made available to manufacturers and NRAs worldwide as soon as possible.

3.4.5 International collaborative study to assess the utility of deep sequencing of virus stocks used in the manufacture of oral poliomyelitis vaccine

The Committee was informed of the outcome of an international collaborative study to investigate the utility of next-generation (deep) sequencing of virus stocks used in the manufacture of live OPV. Currently, the crucial step of ensuring that vaccine strains used in production are appropriately attenuated is carried out using traditional neurovirulence testing in non-human primates and, more recently, in transgenic mice. Loss of attenuation in seed viruses used in production is also monitored by measuring specific nucleotide reversions using the mutant analysis by polymerase chain reaction and restriction enzyme cleavage (MAPREC) test. The Committee was informed that this latter test is a very laborious, technically challenging and requires highly trained staff. The possibility of using deep sequencing was therefore currently being investigated as a suitable alternative since it is simpler, monitors the entire virus genome and is already used in vaccine research and development. It would also allow for monitoring of the whole virus genome for consistency throughout production.

An international collaborative study had therefore been undertaken to validate the utility of deep sequencing as an alternative to the MAPREC test. In Phase 1 of this study, five replicas of each sample were subjected to polymerase chain reaction (PCR) or RNA sequencing using in-house NGS protocols and bioinformatics. The results of this had validated deep sequencing as an alternative to MAPREC for monitoring the 5′ UTR neurovirulence mutation (C instead of U at nucleotide 427) in Sabin type 3 vaccine strains. In Phase 2, the studies had been expanded to cover types 1 and 2 vaccine strains, and to evaluate the genetic consistency of mutational profiles of the entire genome of vaccine viruses. A total of eight laboratories had participated, with three official medicines control laboratories and four manufacturer laboratories in six countries receiving the type 2 vaccine strain.

The results indicated that deep sequencing is indeed highly sensitive and able to detect low-frequency variants in the linear range of raw MAPREC data. Very good correlation was observed between deep sequencing and MAPREC 472C measurements, with deep sequencing results found to be highly repeatable with low within-assay, intra-laboratory and inter-laboratory variability. Deep sequencing measurements were also highly reproducible even when using different methods (RNA, partial PCR or whole-genome PCR) and when the same raw data were analysed using different bioinformatics programmes. Future work will focus on developing the assay validity criteria of sequence coverage, sequence quality and strand bias. Defining the criteria for pass/fail decisions had not yet been finalized and may depend on the development of new reference materials.

The Committee recognized that deep sequencing was potentially a very powerful tool and that the results presented were impressive. The Committee looked forward to hearing more about further developments in this area in due course.

3.4.6 **Revision of the WHO Generic protocol for the calibration of seasonal and pandemic influenza antigen working reagents by WHO essential regulatory laboratories**

The Committee was reminded that influenza antigen reagents are crucial for seasonal and pandemic influenza vaccine production. These reagents are required by manufacturers to measure antigen yields, blend and formulate vaccines, and test final product. The reagents are also required by independent control laboratories for batch release testing. Reagents are produced twice a year by the four ERLs following the recommendations made at each of the biannual WHO influenza vaccine composition meetings. These reagents are required in large amounts and must be produced and calibrated under significant time pressures.

A WHO Generic Protocol was developed in 2011 to harmonize calibration protocols and provide clarity to other stakeholders, primarily vaccine manufacturers. In line with stakeholder requests, ERLs continually work to improve the process – for example, by trialling new technologies for the calibration of the primary liquid standard (PLS). As the protocol is reviewed twice a year at ERL meetings, and given the number of text revisions that have been proposed since 2011, ERLs now consider it timely to update the whole document.

Among the key changes proposed is the addition of a requirement for ERLs to store reagents for secondary calibrations, greater flexibility on the total protein assay, and the addition of alternative methods for the assignment of haemagglutinin (HA) content – such as isotope-dilution mass spectrometry (IDMS). For PLS derived from cell-propagated CVVs the traditional methods have proved problematic and IDMS provides a more robust approach. At their meeting held in January 2018, the ERLs therefore agreed to use IDMS for the calibration of cell-derived PLS. In addition, due to occasional difficulties in obtaining good sheep antisera, greater flexibility is also proposed in the generation of antiserum reagents, including the use of alternative ways of obtaining HA for immunization.

The question was raised of how best to proceed both with the proposed revision of the document and with its future updating. This was in effect a living document and an efficient and rapid way of publishing updates would be useful since ERLs review the document regularly and most changes are minor. If updates were to be published on the GISRS website, then the published protocol would become obsolete and users would need to be alerted to the most up-to-date version. Section 9 of the current published protocol clearly states that it will be reviewed at least annually to ensure that it reflects best practice within ERLs. Crucially, it also already states that any updates to the document will be posted on the GISRS website. The question was also raised regarding the role of the Committee in overseeing the document and its future updates.

The Committee expressed its appreciation for the clear presentation given. Following discussion it was agreed that since there was already a process in place for regularly updating this document – the results of which were posted on the GISRS website as a living document – then the printed version of the document was no longer necessary and should therefore be formally discontinued. It was agreed that significant updates to the document (for example, in critical methodologies) would be presented periodically to the Committee for its information and for its continuing oversight review and comment.

4. International reference materials – antibiotics

All reference materials established at the meeting are listed in Annex 5.

4.1 WHO International Standards and Reference Reagents – antibiotics

4.1.1 Third WHO International Standard for erythromycin

Erythromycin is a mixture of macrolide antibiotics produced by a strain of *Saccharopolyspora erythraea* (formerly known as *Streptomyces erythreus*). It is used to treat a wide range of infections and is on the WHO EML. The international standard for erythromycin is used to calibrate regional and national secondary standards, as well as manufacturers' in-house standards, all of which are routinely used to guarantee the appropriate filling and dosing of erythromycin preparations. There is therefore a global need for this standard.

The Committee was reminded that since stocks of the Second WHO International Standard for erythromycin established in 1978 were running low, and mindful of the issue of widespread and increasing resistance to antibiotics, the Committee had at its meeting in 2017 endorsed a proposal to establish a Third WHO International standard for erythromycin. In response, EDQM as the responsible custodian for the production, establishment and storage of WHO international standards for antibiotics had taken appropriate steps to develop a replacement material. Candidate bulk material donated by a manufacturer had been filled using the same powder-filling process used for the current standard. Vials were filled at a nominal weight of ~75 mg per vial of erythromycin, stoppered under inert gas and sealed. Mean fill weights and relative standard deviations were recorded for each filling session and the identity of the candidate material (EDQM code ISA_65774) confirmed by time-of-flight mass spectrometry. The results obtained were concordant with the expected mass and the candidate material was considered to be suitable for its intended use. Accelerated degradation studies indicated that the proposed candidate material did not exhibit any significant reduction in microbiological potency upon storage at elevated temperatures of up to 50 °C for 6 months. It was therefore concluded that batch stability at the typical storage temperature of -20 °C would be satisfactory.

An international collaborative study involving 15 pharmacopoeial laboratories, NCLs and manufacturer laboratories was undertaken to calibrate the Third WHO International Standard for erythromycin. Study participants were asked to estimate the potency of the candidate material in terms of its microbiological activity against target microorganisms using the diffusion method and the Second WHO International Standard for erythromycin as a reference. Six independent assays were carried out by each participating laboratory and the overall results subjected to statistical analysis.

The Committee considered the report of the study (WHO/BS/2018.2344) together with the stability data generated by EDQM (WHO/BS/2018.2344 – Addendum) and recommended that the candidate material ISA_65774 be established as the Third WHO International Standard for erythromycin with an assigned a potency of 925 IU/mg. The Committee noted that 9488 vials of this international standard were available.

5. International reference materials – blood products and related substances

All reference materials established at the meeting are listed in Annex 5.

5.1 WHO International Standards and Reference Reagents – blood products and related substances

5.1.1 Second WHO International Standard for blood coagulation factor V (plasma, human)

Estimation of blood coagulation factor V clotting activity (FV:C) in human plasma is required for the diagnosis of very rare congenital bleeding disorders and for the investigation of coagulation disorders linked to liver disease. FV:C estimation is also required for the quality control of the therapeutic product.

The First WHO International Standard for factor V (plasma) was established by the Committee in 2005 with a single assigned value of 0.74 IU/ampoule for FV:C. Approximately 300–400 ampoules have since been issued annually and the remaining stocks will be exhausted within a year. An international collaborative study was therefore conducted involving 30 laboratories from 14 countries to value assign a candidate material (NIBSC code 16/374) proposed for use as the Second WHO International Standard for blood coagulation factor V (plasma, human).

Estimation of FV:C for the candidate material calculated relative to the current WHO international standard resulted in an overall mean value of 0.72 IU/ml (n = 34), with low inter-laboratory variability observed (geometric coefficient of variation (GCV) = 3.19%). An identical mean value was obtained relative to local normal plasma pools indicating that the relationship of the IU to normal plasma had been maintained. This was further supported by estimates made of local normal plasma pools relative to the current WHO international standard which returned an overall mean of 1.00 IU/ml (n = 32). Such low inter-laboratory variability and complete agreement between estimates relative to both the current WHO international standard and local normal pools is consistent with robust correlation between the IU value of the current WHO international standard and that of the candidate material 16/374.

Estimates were also made of the FV antigen (FV:Ag) value of the candidate material. Five datasets from four laboratories (18 assays in total) were received, with the candidate material included as coded duplicates in each assay to provide a total of 36 estimates for the new value assignment. Estimates were calculated relative to local normal plasma pools using an arbitrary value of 1.00 unit/ml for each pool. The combined results produced an overall mean of 0.75 units/ml (inter-laboratory GCV = 7.26%). Upon establishment of the antigen value to the proposed WHO international standard the "unit" will be replaced by "IU".

An accelerated degradation study was carried out to evaluate the stability of the candidate material. The predicted loss of potency in ampoules stored at the bulk storage temperature of −20 °C was estimated to be less than 0.1% per year for clotting activity and antigen. This was considered to be consistent with suitable stability for the proposed standard. Further stability testing will take place during the lifetime of the standard.

The Committee considered the report of the study (WHO/BS/2018.2341) and recommended that the candidate material 16/374 be established as the Second WHO International Standard for blood coagulation factor V (plasma, human), with assigned unitages of 0.72 IU/ampoule for FV:C relative to the First WHO International Standard for factor V (plasma) and 0.75 IU/ampoule for FV:Ag relative to local normal pools.

5.1.2 **Third WHO International Standard for anti-D immunoglobulin (human)**

Anti-D immunoglobulin is used worldwide for the prevention of haemolytic disease in newborns and its clinical use requires estimation of its potency against a reference preparation. In the 1970s, WHO and CBER independently established reference standards for anti-D immunoglobulin to ensure that appropriate potency requirements were met. Subsequent concerns over contamination with hepatitis C virus RNA and dwindling stocks led to the establishment of the Second WHO International Standard for anti-D immunoglobulin in 2003. Stocks of this new "global" standard were shared between CBER, EDQM and NIBSC for distribution and were now almost depleted.

Two candidate materials (NIBSC codes 16/278 and 16/332) along with other study samples had therefore been evaluated and calibrated against the current WHO international standard in an international collaborative study involving 21 laboratories in 15 countries. With one exception, all of the laboratories used autoanalyser, competitive enzyme immunoassay and/or flow cytometry methodologies. The overall geometric mean potency of the candidate material 16/332 was 296.6 IU/ampoule (inter-laboratory GCV = 4.7%). Analysis of the immunoglobulin preparations using size-exclusion high-performance liquid chromatography (SE–HPLC) demonstrated combined monomeric and dimeric IgG peak areas of > 95% for all samples. Accelerated stability studies indicated a predicted loss of potency per year of < 0.001% for 16/278 when stored at −20 °C. For the candidate material 16/332, loss of potency was only measurable at 56 °C indicating that the material would be stable for decades when stored at −20 °C. In addition, the potency results obtained for 16/332 exhibited the least inter-laboratory and inter-assay variability.

The Committee noted that the autoanalyser results appeared to be significantly higher than those obtained using either competitive enzyme immunoassay or flow cytometry – raising the question of the validity of results obtained using the autoanalyser method. It was pointed out that only one of the test values was significantly higher than the other values recorded and that this had not impacted on the overall analysis. Moreover, the majority of autoanalyser results were well within the same margins obtained using the other methods. It was further pointed out that although the autoanalyser method is somewhat sensitive to matrix effects when used with antibodies, these effects are not significant. The Committee considered the report of the study (WHO/BS/2018.2332) and recommended that the candidate material 16/332 be established as the Third WHO International Standard for anti-D immunoglobulin with an assigned unitage of 297 IU/ampoule.

5.2 Proposed new projects and updates – blood products and related substances

5.2.1 Proposed First WHO International Standard for unfractionated heparin for molecular weight calibration

Currently there are two pharmacopoeial standards for the molecular weight calibration of unfractionated heparin and it is unclear whether these two standards are traceable to each other. A higher-order WHO standard was now required to ensure the harmonization of molecular weight measurements of unfractionated heparin products. It was proposed that evaluation of a new standard would be conducted in three phases. In Phase 1, an in-house study would be carried out to identify a suitable candidate material. This study may require the blending of different heparin active pharmaceutical ingredients to obtain the molecular weight profile required to cover the wide range of unfractionated heparin products available. To ensure continuity of the molecular weight scale, the proposed candidate material would be compared to the currently used pharmacopoeial standards. In Phase 2, an international collaborative study would be conducted to further assess the candidate material and to allow for the calculation of a molecular weight table. The table would then be used to calibrate the molecular weight of a number of unknown unfractionated heparin samples. In Phase 3, a further international collaborative study would be conducted to assess the fitness for purpose of the proposed international standard. This would involve using the molecular weight table produced in Phase 2 to measure the molecular weights of several common unfractionated heparin samples. Each participant laboratory would also assess a number of representative in-house unfractionated heparin preparations. It was envisaged that suitable candidate material would be obtained by early 2019. The conducting of the Phase 1–3 studies between March 2019 and June 2020 would allow for the submission of a proposal to the Committee in 2020 to establish the new WHO international standard.

During discussion the issue was raised of the intended users of the new standard given the availability of the current standards in China and the USA. It was pointed out that the new WHO international standard would allow for comparison of the two available standards and for the replacement of the complex pharmacopoeial methods currently used. Discussion then turned to the more general issue of the process by which this proposal had come to the Committee. It was noted that this item had not been discussed during the meeting of the WHO network of collaborating centres for blood products and in vitro diagnostics earlier in the year and that consideration might usefully be given to how best to facilitate the timely development and discussion of such proposals. After due consideration, the Committee endorsed the proposal (WHO/BS/2018.2342) to develop a First WHO International Standard for unfractionated heparin for molecular weight calibration.

5.2.2 Proposed Third WHO International Standard for von Willebrand factor concentrate

Von Willebrand factor (VWF) concentrates are used as a replacement therapy in the bleeding disorder von Willebrand disease – the most common bleeding disorder in humans. Some subtypes of the disease can only be treated using purified concentrates. Ensuring effective and safe dosage relies on potency labelling relative to the WHO international standard. Use of the standard also supports the global harmonization of product potency labelling.

The standard is in high demand (800–900 ampoules per annum) and stocks of the current second WHO international standard will be exhausted in 2–3 years and are thus in need of replacement. The collection of suitable candidate materials was now under way, with filling and characterization scheduled to take place in 2019 followed by an international collaborative study. It was envisaged that the results of the study would then be submitted to the Committee for its consideration in 2020.

It was noted during discussion that two new test methods had been developed since the establishment of the current WHO international standard, and that these were increasingly being used. This raised the issue of ensuring continuity given the possibility that the new methods might measure different aspects of activity compared to the earlier assays. It was clarified that although the new methods were integrated into the collaborative study, the results they gave would only be used in the calibration of the candidate material if they did not deviate from those obtained using the original methods. The question was also raised of whether a plasma-derived international standard would be commutable with recombinant products. It was agreed that if available, recombinant VWF products would be included in the collaborative study to specifically test this aspect. The Committee endorsed the proposal (WHO/BS/2018.2342) to develop a Third WHO International Standard for von Willebrand factor concentrate.

5.2.3 Update on the WHO snakebite antivenom project

The Committee was provided with an update on recent progress made in the assessment of antivenoms intended for use in sub-Saharan Africa. This WHO project had started in December 2015 with a call to manufacturers to submit potentially suitable products for evaluation. Nine applications were received; two of which were rejected due to regional unsuitability and two due to dossier deficiencies. The remaining five products were sent for laboratory investigation of their physicochemical properties and specific venom immunorecognition. Potency testing and quantitative antivenomics studies had now been completed and technical reports were being prepared for manufacturers. GMP inspections had also been conducted in applicant facilities and a number of issues identified, including numerous critical and major findings. To improve local understanding of GMP requirements, a call for corrective and preventive actions had been issued and response actions are being undertaken. Follow-up inspections may be required to verify compliance with the improvement process prior to the issuing of final recommendations. Some manufacturers had already reported good progress towards compliance with the programme, the aim of which is to support manufacturers in the production of safe and efficacious antivenoms.

Strong support, led by Costa Rica, continues to be expressed by Member States for the programme. In May 2018, resolution WHA71.5 on snakebite envenoming was adopted by the Seventy-first World Health Assembly and a draft roadmap prepared. This roadmap is now being reviewed at WHO regional office level with a view to publication in early 2019 followed by a stakeholder meeting to mobilize support. WHO will continue to advocate for this issue and to identify resources to allow for implementation of the roadmap.

Future needs and possible next steps for the programme include the development of specific standards for different snake species in different parts of the world. In addition to antivenom assessment, consideration was also being given to developing an antivenom prequalification procedure. The standardization and optimization of antivenom production processes and the raising of manufacturing standards were viewed as key areas. Efforts are also needed to develop immunization schedules, adjuvant technologies and other approaches to increase the specific immune response to poorly antigenic toxins.

In order to make the best use of available resources it will be crucially important to harness synergies between WHOCCs at global and regional level. The example was given of work now under way to develop snake antivenom standards at the University of Melbourne. The university is also expected to participate in the generation of written standards and is on the way to acquiring WHOCC status. Updating of the WHO snake antivenom database is also planned, with known manufacturers of antivenom to be included whether or not they are involved in the WHO assessment scheme. WHO will also monitor and review research to develop innovative new technologies for producing medicines against snakebites.

During discussion, an update was requested of the progress made in conferring WHOCC status on the University of Melbourne, and clarification of whether it would then become part of the WHO network of collaborating centres for blood products and in vitro diagnostics. While this would appear to be a reasonable step there seemed to be little overlap between these areas and the manufacture of antivenoms. Given the lack of progress since the first sub-Saharan workshop on this subject a decade ago, the current momentum in this field was very much welcomed. At present, relevant regulatory knowledge and experience are severely limited, with an ongoing lack of awareness of treatment options. There was however broad recognition of the complexities in this area. Given that snake venom is a highly complex and geographically variable mixture of proteins, cross-protection conferred by antivenoms against the identified main toxic components was likely to be of key importance. The Committee noted the progress that had been made and expressed its strong support for the continuation of the programme.

6. International reference materials – cellular and gene therapies

All reference materials established at the meeting are listed in Annex 5.

6.1 Proposed new projects and updates – cellular and gene therapies

6.1.1 Proposed First WHO International Reference Reagent for mesenchymal stromal cell identity for flow cytometry

One of the fastest growing areas in the field of cellular therapies is the use of human multipotent mesenchymal stromal cells (MSCs) for clinical application. More than 150 studies involving the use of MSCs have now been completed, with 67 clinical trials currently under way and a further 184 actively recruiting. The international scientific community has agreed upon a number of minimal cell characteristics that define MSCs. Part of this characterization requires the assessment of a panel of markers using flow cytometry. MSCs are positive for CD73, CD90 and CD105 and negative for CD34, CD45, CD11b, CD19 and HLA Class II.

Currently there are no international reference preparations for MSCs used for advanced therapies, and a degree of disarray exists within the field in the characterization and testing used to define MSC populations. Following calls from the scientific community, a proposal had been made to develop a WHO international reference reagent for MSC identity for flow cytometry derived from human pluripotent stem cells. It is intended that this standard will fulfil the MSC signature characteristics described above and will be validated against primary MSCs. The proposed reference reagent is intended to be used during flow cytometry identity assessment of MSC products and will facilitate validation and verification of the identity of MSC populations used in clinical applications. The provision of such a reference reagent will also allow for assessment of batch-to-batch consistency and aid in the harmonization of cell-based therapies.

A collaborative study will be conducted to evaluate a candidate material using a variety of flow cytometers, antibodies and protocols, while comparing it with different in vivo and in vitro MSC source materials. The quantitative data derived from the collaborative study would then be used to establish a consensus gene-expression range for each gene included in the MSC signature. The Committee was informed that the generation of MSCs from human pluripotent stem cells had now been completed, with bulk cell culture, quality control and filling activities scheduled to follow in 2019. Following data analysis, the study results obtained for the candidate material were scheduled for submission to the Committee for its consideration in 2020. Current data demonstrate that the freeze-dried cells are stable for up to 12 months but a master cell bank is kept to ensure a continuous supply.

The Committee considered this to be an interesting proposal but it would be important to make it very clear that the reference material would not be a potency or quantitative standard. Rather, it would be intended for use in characterizing the surface phenotype of cells used in clinical studies – even though it is not certain if the markers chosen are therapeutically significant. However, the batch-to-batch consistency of cells used in clinical studies could be monitored using the proposed reagent. The Committee endorsed the proposal (WHO/BS/2018.2342) to develop a First WHO International Reference Reagent for mesenchymal stromal cell identity for flow cytometry.

7. International reference materials – in vitro diagnostics

All reference materials established at the meeting are listed in Annex 5.

7.1 WHO International Standards and Reference Reagents – in vitro diagnostics

7.1.1 First WHO International Reference Reagent for CD4+ T-cells (human)

Untreated HIV infection typically leads to the loss of CD4+ T-cells required to mount an effective immune response against infections. The baseline measurement of CD4+ T-cell counts in patients entering or re-entering treatment is thus vital in the assessment of HIV disease progression. Following the initiation of antiretroviral treatment, CD4+ T-cell count can also be monitored to evaluate therapeutic response. However, there is a lack of harmonization in CD4+ T-cell counting which has been highlighted by WHO as an issue in patient care. To help improve the international harmonization of CD4+ T-cell counting, the Committee at its meeting in 2010 endorsed a proposal to develop a WHO international reference reagent to serve as a standard for CD4+ T-cell counting methods.

An international study had now been conducted to develop and evaluate a freeze-dried candidate material (NIBSC code 15/270) for use as a reference reagent for CD4+ T-cell enumeration technologies. This material had been prepared from pooled human blood leukocytes isolated from donations to the United Kingdom National Blood Service and tested for a range of viral infections. All virology results were negative. The cells were suspended in a freeze-drying formulation, distributed into glass ampoules, freeze-dried and sealed under nitrogen. Studies indicated satisfactory stability at −20 °C storage. Although the material will require a cold chain for transport this is not a significant issue as it is intended for use mainly by manufacturers. The material was evaluated by 12 laboratories from eight countries in four WHO regions. The participating laboratories used different CD4+ T-cell counting technologies, all of which had been deemed to be suitable on the basis of independent peer-reviewed data. The methods used included single-platform and dual-platform flow cytometry, dedicated CD4+ systems and point-of-care technologies.

Results indicated that the candidate material 15/270 worked well in flow cytometry platforms and with the point-of-care technologies tested but could not be read by the dedicated CD4+ systems BD FACS Count and BD FACS Presto. Unfortunately the study had been unable to cover of all the technologies used for CD4+ T-cell counting and it will be important to test the material in the point-of-care device Alere Pima – a CD4+ T-cell test commonly used in sub-Saharan Africa. The candidate material was also found to be incompatible with one of the commercial lysis reagents used and red blood cell lysis reagents will need to be independently evaluated in each centre to determine suitability. Participants had been asked to express the CD4+ T-cell concentrations found as both number of CD4+ T-cells per µl and as a percentage of total white blood cells, when applicable to their routine method. An overall mean value and standard deviation was calculated for the candidate material and a normal distribution was extrapolated.

Extensive discussion took place regarding the appropriate assignment of a unit and the reality of what this will offer given the wide acceptable range due to the extrapolated normal distribution. It was suggested that provision of this range may be misleading for laboratories and send out the wrong message in relation to acceptable level of variability. Typically, laboratories would be expected to achieve coefficients of variation of < 10% yet the mean value observed in this study was 16%. It was clarified that the range observed within laboratories was narrower than the overall study value and one function of the candidate material would be to give laboratories an insight into their own performance.

The issue of testing in LMIC was also discussed and clarification requested of the number of assays used in the study that had been prequalified by the WHO IVD Prequalification Team. It was noted that the Alere Pima CD4+ T-cell test had been prequalified in 2012 and agreement was reached that further work would be carried out to better understand the suitability of the candidate material for use in this test. There was also discussion of the compatibility of some red blood cell lysis reagents with the candidate material. As only one brand of lysis reagent had appeared to be problematic, it was advised that this should be specifically notified in the instructions for use (IFU). Among the other restrictions to be clearly outlined in the IFU was the indication that the material is not suitable for the calibration of CD4+ T-cell counting systems.

The Committee considered the report of the study (WHO/BS/2018.2333) and recommended that the candidate material 15/270 be established as the First WHO International Reference Reagent for CD4+ T-cells (human). It was agreed that the availability of this WHO international reference reagent would benefit the majority of users of CD4+ T-cell counting technologies, improve testing quality and positively impact on patient treatment. As the direct assignment of a value was considered potentially confusing, the range obtained in the collaborative study should instead be outlined in the IFU as part of the intended application of the material and the expected performance range within individual laboratories made clear. Further action points agreed included WHO internal liaison to promote the use of the material in LMIC including through the provision of education to end users, assessment of the use of the international reference reagent in the Pima test and further investigation of the reasons for no result being returned by particular assays.

7.1.2 First WHO International Reference Panel for HIV-1 p24 antigen and First WHO International Reference Reagent for HIV-2 p26 antigen

The characterization of HIV-1 strains has resulted in the identification of four distinct groups – namely: M (major) consisting of subtypes A–K, and the more uncommon groups N, O and P. In addition, the global distribution of subtypes A–K is not static, with HIV strains spreading with ease between geographical regions. For example, in Western Europe, subtype B previously dominated but following population movements a number of non-B subtypes are becoming more prevalent. This is leading to recombination events within the dually infected and associated increases in the number of circulating and unique recombinant forms (CRFs and URFs respectively). In such a dynamic and complex situation, increasingly sensitive HIV diagnostics and viral load assays are required.

NAT-based assays remain the most sensitive and accurate diagnostic technology used, with RNA detectable 12 days after infection. However, such assays are also expensive and require dedicated infrastructure, equipment and expertise which may not be available in LMIC. As these methods are also time consuming and slow to perform, both antigen-only and fourth-generation antigen/antibody (Ag/Ab) combination immunoassays still play an important role in public health. Such assays are used to detect the core HIV-1 capsid protein p24, which is a good indicator of HIV-1 infection since free p24 in the blood is present and elevated in the early stages of infection before an immune response can be established. Immunoassays are low-cost by comparison to NAT-based assays and can be performed in resource-poor settings using generic equipment such as universal washers and spectrometers. This is particularly evident in the case of rapid test systems or point-of-care technologies which tend to be portable and can be taken to the patient.

The Committee was informed that a study had been undertaken using a large subtype panel of virus-like particles (VLPs) containing the HIV *Gag-pr* region from clinical samples. This study had revealed large variations in the ability of currently used HIV immunoassays to detect certain subtypes or CRFs with some assays giving false-negative results or exhibiting reduced sensitivity for non-subtype B samples. Following discussions between NIBSC and the study group, a proposal was made to investigate the suitability of the study VLPs to act as international reference materials. After establishing the suitability of a lyophilized VLP in a small pilot study, a proposal had been made to the Committee in 2015 to proceed with the establishment of two WHO international reference preparations – one for HIV-1 p24 and one for HIV-2 p26. Following endorsement by the Committee, a panel of 12 HIV-1 subtypes/CRF VLPs and a single HIV-2 VLP were selected from the larger study panel and evaluated in an international collaborative study.

Fifteen laboratories returned data, with some laboratories testing the panel in more than one assay. A total of 25 datasets were received – 20 for Ag/Ab combination assays, four for antigen-only assays and one for a rapid test/point-of-care assay. Results indicated a number of assay weaknesses in relation to some of the panel members – notably the Bio-Rad Access which showed low specificity and sensitivity to a majority of the samples, and three Biomerieux assays which could not detect the subtype C or D samples. Overall, the candidate materials intended for use in HIV-1 p24 antigen assays showed parallelism to the current WHO International Reference Reagent for HIV-1 p24 antigen established in 1992. This raised the possibility of formally assigning a potency expressed in IU to each of the HIV-1 panel members for inclusion as a table the IFU. Due to the variability observed between assays for the HIV-2 candidate material no proposal was made to assign potency.

The Committee acknowledged the extensive efforts made in characterizing and assessing the candidate materials and agreed on the necessity for an HIV-1 p24 reference panel. Due to the prior establishment of the current international reference reagent it was not considered appropriate to assign IU values to the panel members without the assignment of uncertainty of measurement estimates. Metrologically speaking, this would constitute the formulation of secondary materials and was not part of the remit of the Committee. A suggestion to assign a unit value to the materials, instead of IU, was also rejected on the grounds that the international guidelines to which the manufacturers of these assays conform reference the use of IU. The Committee considered the report of the study (WHO/BS/2018.2334) and recommended that the HIV-1 panel members be established as the First WHO International Reference Panel for HIV-1 p24 antigen. The Committee agreed that no unit should be formally assigned to any panel member but that the calibrated values obtained from the study should be made available in a table in the IFU. The Committee further recommended that the HIV-2 candidate material be established as the First WHO International Reference Reagent for HIV-2 p26 antigen with no unit assignment.

7.1.3 First WHO International Reference Reagent for von Willebrand factor (plasma) binding to recombinant glycoprotein Ib

Diagnosis of the bleeding disorder von Willebrand disease includes measurement of VWF binding to the glycoprotein Ib (GPIb) receptor on the platelet surface. The ristocetin cofactor method originally used to measure this activity is associated with large variability and poor sensitivity. In recent years, alternative methods have been developed based on the binding of VWF to recombinant GPIb. These methods either rely on the presence of ristocetin for VWF binding (VWF:GPIbR) or employ a "gain-of-function" mutant of GPIb which does not require ristocetin for VWF binding (VWF:GPIbM). Increasing use of these new methods has led to an urgent need for their standardization at the international level in order to support the harmonization of test results and prevent potential divergence between laboratories should locally derived units be used.

Following discussions within the VWF sub-committee of the International Society on Thrombosis and Haemostasis (ISTH) it was agreed that a proposal be made to the Committee to assign the value of 0.87 IU/ampoule currently used for the VWF ristocetin cofactor method (VWF:RCo) in the Sixth WHO International Standard for blood coagulation factor VIII and von Willebrand factor (plasma) as the "units" of the proposed First WHO International Reference Reagent for von Willebrand factor (plasma) binding to recombinant glycoprotein Ib. The Sixth WHO International Standard for blood coagulation factor VIII and von Willebrand factor (plasma) would then serve as this proposed WHO international reference reagent. This proposal had formally been endorsed by the ISTH Scientific and Standardization Committee in July 2018. This retrospective approach to establish the proposed international reference reagent was not based on collaborative studies but was supported by the results of an independent study published in 2018. Rather than be replaced, the current WHO international standard will also serve as the international reference reagent for the new methods, thus avoiding the development of different standards for an identical analyte.

It was further proposed that the envisaged replacement of the current sixth WHO international standard in approximately two years be used as an opportunity to value assign the replacement seventh WHO international standard for VWF:RCo, VWF:GPIbM and VWF:GPIbR methods by assay relative to the current international standard, and to review the link with local normal plasma pools. The establishment of the seventh WHO international standard could also be used to change the status of the VWF:GPIbM and VWF:GPIbR units to IU. It was emphasized that assigned values for VWF:RCo on secondary standards should not be used for calculating VWF:GPIbM and VWF:GPIbR results. Secondary standards should instead be calibrated for VWF:GPIbM and VWF:GPIbR by assay relative to the sixth WHO international standard.

The Committee considered the report of the study (WHO/BS/2018.2337) and recommended that the Sixth WHO International Standard for blood coagulation factor VIII and von Willebrand factor (plasma) be established as the First WHO International Reference Reagent for von Willebrand factor (plasma) binding to recombinant glycoprotein Ib with the assigned value of 0.87 u/ampoule for use in both VWF:GPIbM and VWF:GPIbR assays. The Committee noted the opportunity that will be provided during the replacement of the current sixth WHO international standard in approximately two years to effect the further changes proposed above.

7.1.4 Second WHO International Standard for prostate specific antigen (free) and Second WHO International Standard for prostate specific antigen (human) (total: PSA-ACT + free PSA)

Prostate specific antigen (PSA) is a 28.4 kDa kallikrein-related peptidase with a physiological role in liquefying seminal fluid. Clinically, both free PSA (fPSA) and total PSA in serum are measured by immunoassays for the purposes of diagnosing and monitoring the treatment of prostate cancers. Stocks of the current first WHO international standards used for the calibration of immunoassays are almost exhausted and in 2014 the Committee recognized the need for replacement international standards to be developed.

A candidate material (NIBSC code 17/102) was evaluated for its suitability to serve as an international standard for use in fPSA immunoassays in an international collaborative study involving 10 laboratories in eight countries. A second candidate material (NIBSC code 17/100) was separately evaluated for use as an international standard for total PSA (PSA-ACT + free PSA) in an international collaborative study involving the same 10 laboratories.

The geometric mean of the laboratory estimates for the fPSA content of the current international standard (NIBSC code 96/668) agreed with its originally assigned value of 1 µg/vial, with a corresponding geometric mean value of 0.545 µg/ampoule obtained for the candidate material 17/102 (95% CI = 0.508–0.586; n = 21; GCV = 17.0%) with a robust mean of 0.533 µg/ampoule. These and other data would support a value assignment of 0.53 µg/ampoule. An assessment of the impact of the proposed new international standard on the routine measurement of fPSA in human serum samples indicated its suitability for the continued calibration of immunoassay methods. On the basis of an accelerated degradation study, the candidate material 17/102 would also appear to be sufficiently stable to serve as an international standard.

The geometric mean of the laboratory estimates for the total PSA content of the current international standard (NIBSC code 96/670) also agreed with its originally assigned value of 1 µg/vial, with a corresponding geometric mean value of 0.514 µg/ampoule obtained for the candidate material 17/100 (95% CI = 0.489–0.542; n = 22; GCV = 12.3%) with a robust mean of 0.505 µg/ampoule. These and other data would support a value assignment of 0.5 µg/ampoule. Laboratory estimates of the free PSA content of 17/100, determined as a percentage of the corresponding total PSA estimate for each method, was 12.1% which was comparable to that of 96/670 (12.7%). An assessment of the impact of the proposed new international standard on the routine measurement of total PSA in human serum samples indicated its suitability for the continued calibration of immunoassay methods. On the basis of an accelerated degradation study, the candidate material 17/100 would also appear to be sufficiently stable to serve as an international standard.

During discussion it was clarified that the fPSA commutability data presented were not the result of a complete commutability study, which had not been the intention. The aim was to demonstrate that the candidate material did not deviate from the former reference material in order to maintain the status quo, and to show comparability rather than commutability. The limits used in the study were also statistically defined (two standard deviations) and were not necessarily clinically relevant. The use of those assays in which commutability was found to be inconclusive may therefore still be acceptable.

The Committee considered the reports of the studies (WHO/BS/2018.2339 and WHO/BS/2018.2340) and recommended that: (a) the candidate material 17/102 be established as the Second WHO International Standard for prostate specific antigen (free) with an assigned content of 0.53 µg/ampoule; and (b) the candidate material 17/100 be established as the Second WHO International Standard for prostate specific antigen (human) (total: PSA-ACT + free PSA) with an assigned content of 0.50 µg/ampoule.

7.1.5   Second WHO International Standard for HIV-2 RNA for NAT-based assays

HIV-2 was first isolated in 1986 by the Paris Pasteur Institute from an endemic region in West Africa. Since then, nine distinct lineages (A–I) have been isolated. In addition to West Africa, HIV-2 is found mainly in former Portuguese colonies, Portugal and France with evidence suggesting its decreasing prevalence. HIV-2 is associated with lower rates of transmission and progression to acquired immune deficiency syndrome, with patients demonstrating higher CD4+ T-cell counts and lower viral loads compared to patients infected with HIV-1. Although pathology appears similar, there are significant differences observed in the immune system response to infection with HIV-2. Because not all treatments established for HIV-1 are effective against HIV-2, the accurate and timely diagnosis of HIV-2 infection is vital to ensure that the correct therapy can be given and that individuals can be informed of their infection status to reduce the risk of unintended transmission. Although screening for HIV-2 RNA is not mandated in as many countries as it is for HIV-1, accurate and sensitive assays are also crucially important in ensuring a safe blood supply in countries where HIV-2 is prevalent.

NAT-based assays are the most widely used and most sensitive method for the detection and quantification of HIV-2 RNA in human serum and plasma, and a range of commercial and laboratory-developed assays are in use. As such assays are routinely used to manage HIV infections, and there remains a risk of transfusion-transmitted infection due to window-period donations, there is an ongoing need for their standardization.

Following the establishment of the First WHO International Standard for HIV-2 RNA in 2009 with an assigned potency of 1000 IU/ml many users indicated that the titre was too low for calibration purposes. It had therefore been proposed that a replacement material be formulated at a higher titre (~10^6 IU/ml). The standard will be used to calibrate secondary standards for the onward calibration of HIV-2 NAT-based assays. Envisaged users include diagnostic kit manufacturers, blood fractionators, reference laboratories, diagnostics laboratories, providers of external quality assessment and official medicines control laboratories.

The proposed freeze-dried candidate material (NIBSC code 16/296) and its liquid bulk equivalent were evaluated in an international collaborative study involving 15 laboratories from 11 countries. Parallel evaluations were also made of the current first international standard, an HIV-2 working reagent and a clinical specimen of HIV-2-positive plasma. The candidate material was prepared from the same HIV-2 subtype A strain used to produce the first international standard, with the complete genome sequence previously determined by Sanger sequencing. A variety of qualitative and quantitative assays were used, with the qualitative assays being mostly commercial and the quantitative assays predominantly laboratory developed (and exhibiting greater variability). Agreement between laboratories was improved when the potencies of high-titre samples were expressed relative to the current and candidate reference materials – an effect not observed for all low-titre sample potencies. The overall mean reported estimates for the candidate material using qualitative assays was 5.26 $\log_{10}$ NAT-detectable units/ml and 5.40 $\log_{10}$ IU/ml using quantitative assays, with standard deviations of 0.28 and 0.32 respectively. The mean estimate across both qualitative and quantitative assays was 5.46 $\log_{10}$ IU/ml when expressed relative to the current standard. Inter-laboratory variation was on the whole greater than intra-laboratory variation. Accelerated degradation at 10 months indicated minimal loss in potency when stored at $-20\,°C$. Results from further time points of the extended stability study were expected to yield a more reliable stability prediction using the Arrhenius model.

The Committee considered the report of the study (WHO/BS/2018.2343) and recommended that the candidate material 16/296 be established as the Second WHO International Standard for HIV-2 RNA for NAT-based assays with an assigned value of 1.44 x 10^5 IU/vial.

7.1.6   First WHO International Standard for adenovirus DNA for NAT-based assays

Human adenoviruses (HAdVs) are non-enveloped DNA viruses comprising 70 types grouped into seven species (HAdV-A–HAdV-G). Most HAdV species circulate globally with predominant types differing geographically. Primary infection occurs in young children via multiple transmission routes. HAdVs cause a range of usually self-limiting diseases in immunocompetent individuals – including conjunctivitis, gastroenteritis, hepatitis, myocarditis and pneumonia. However, they can cause significant morbidity and mortality in the immunocompromised, particularly haematopoietic stem cell patients.

NAT-based assays such as real-time PCR are typically used for the diagnosis and monitoring of HAdV infections. Given the known correlation between high viral loads in peripheral blood and the risk of invasive disease and mortality in transplant recipients, the prospective monitoring of HAdV viral load in whole blood or plasma is recommended in the transplant setting to guide the initiation of therapy and monitor response. Additionally, there is increasing evidence that the PCR monitoring of stool samples from paediatric haematopoietic stem cell patients can provide early prognostic information. The effective monitoring of infection in immunocompromised patients thus depends upon the reliable quantification of all relevant HAdV types in different clinical specimens. A number of commercial HAdV assays are available which typically target conserved regions of the HAdV genome. However, there is a lack of data on performance variability among different NAT-based assays and on the effectiveness of quantification of different HAdV types.

In 2006, a pilot collaborative study was conducted to investigate the inter- and intra-laboratory variability of HAdV DNA quantification using a number of different NAT-based assays. Assay performance was investigated using a panel of samples representing nine HAdV types. Inter-laboratory variability was found to be significantly higher than intra-laboratory variability for the testing of both cultured virus and patient samples, highlighting a clear need for the standardization of HAdV NAT assays. The results of this study and of a subsequent 2016 pilot study were used to guide the selection and formulation of source materials for evaluation as candidate reference materials for use in the standardization of HAdV NAT-based assays.

An international collaborative study was conducted involving 32 laboratories in 13 countries. Study participants were asked to evaluate the suitability of two lyophilized HAdV type 2 candidate materials (NIBSC codes 16/306 and 16/324) using their own routine HAdV NAT-based assay. The candidate materials were evaluated alongside three laboratory-grown viruses and three clinical isolates of different HAdV types. A wide range of HAdV NAT-based assays were used in the evaluation, the majority of which were quantitative real-time PCR assays targeting the hexon protein gene. For all samples, inter-laboratory variation was significantly greater than the intra-laboratory variation. Harmonization of HAdV DNA measurements for the virus cultures was observed when the mean estimates were expressed relative to the two candidate materials, with the greatest degree harmonization observed when samples were matched by HAdV type or species. For the clinical isolates, there was also some improvement in inter-laboratory agreement. Ongoing accelerated thermal degradation studies at one year indicate that both candidate materials are stable and suitable for long-term use. It was pointed out that the type 2 virus used in candidate material 16/324 is widely used as a common reference strain. It was further highlighted that a statement would be added in the IFU to reflect the limited opportunity to assess commutability, particularly in non-C species adenoviruses.

The Committee considered the report of the study (WHO/BS/2018.2346) and recommended that the candidate material 16/324 be established as the First WHO International Standard for adenovirus DNA for NAT-based assays with a value of 2×10^8 IU/vial.

7.2 Proposed new projects and updates – in vitro diagnostics

7.2.1 Proposed additional WHO international reference reagents for blood group genotyping

The genotyping of blood group has become a common practice to overcome a number of issues associated with conventional serological assays, which include: (a) a lack of serological reagents; (b) poor reliability or scarcity of serological reagents; (c) resolving complex cases of red blood cell phenotyping when patients have been multiply transfused; (d) predicting red blood cell phenotype when patients have a positive direct antiglobulin test; (e) determination of RHD zygosity, which is important for predicting fetal D status from D-alloimmunized pregnant mothers using non-invasive testing; and (f) reagent typing discrepancies.

The Committee was informed that CBER had developed a blood group genotyping panel for institutional use comprising 18 lyophilized genomic DNA samples from phenotyped donors. These samples represent 40 genetic markers generating red blood cell antigenic polymorphisms associated with 17 blood group systems. However, there are already four current WHO international reference reagents for blood group genotyping, established in 2011. The current proposal was not intended to replace these existing reference reagents but to add the CBER materials, thus increasing the number of reference reagent resources to 22. This will expand the number of red blood cell polymorphisms currently represented in the WHO reference reagents for blood group genotyping. Although there is some overlap in terms of common alleles already represented in three of the existing WHO reference reagents, these overlapping alleles have been characterized using a range of advanced technique not available during the development of the current reagent set. Anticipated users include laboratories performing genotyping, test kit manufacturers and regulatory agencies. The material is suitable for use as controls, to assist assay development and for the validation of assays and testing methods.

The study to develop the panel was an independent CBER initiative involving multiple steps, including ethical approval for research using human samples, donor recruitment, sample collection and testing, and analysis of test results. Stability and accelerated degradation studies were also performed. In a

WHO Technical Report Series, No. 1016, 2019

wider collaborative study, 28 laboratories in 13 countries from North and South America, Europe, Asia, Middle East, and Australia. Two laboratories provided 30 datasets using a wide variety of genotyping techniques. Study data were then analyzed and a full report prepared for the Committee in support of the proposed project to add the 18 CBER reference reagents to the existing set of WHO international reference reagents. The additional reference reagents would be provided independently with both sets circulated despite the overlap of three members. In both cases, reagents could either be distributed as a requested panel or as individual reagents depending on the end user needs.

The Committee endorsed the proposal (WHO/BS/2018.2342) to develop a set of 18 additional WHO international reference reagents for blood group genotyping. The existing WHO international reference reagents would continue to be distributed as a set or individually. It was envisaged that prior to the formal establishment of the additional reference reagents, further discussion would be required to clarify the issue of nomenclature in cases where the expansion of existing reference reagents or panels was being proposed – an issue not confined to these materials.

7.2.2 Proposed First WHO international standards for (cell line name) cancer genomes

The Committee was reminded of its endorsement in 2017 of a proposal to develop a First WHO International Reference Panel for cancer mutation detection. Endorsement was now being sought for a proposal to instead develop individual WHO international standards for cancer genomes in place of the originally proposed WHO panel. This would involve the initiation of a cancer genomic standards programme in which a common approach would be used to develop multiple standards – thus increasing the coverage of clinically relevant genomes and allowing for timely alignment with the development of multiple anti-cancer drugs targeted to tumour biomarkers. The development of WHO international standards would also assist in the development of NGS for multiple marker detection and quantification in tumour DNA, as this technology is becoming increasingly affordable and accessible.

It was proposed that in the first instance the standards developed would comprise three genomic DNAs, each obtained from a single cell line, and five clinically relevant variants as follows:

- ATDC101 (colon adenocarcinoma): *PIK3CA* p.E545K;
- ATDC102 (leukaemia): *TP53* p.R306*, *NRAS* p.G12C, *PTEN* p.K267fs*9, *MAP2K1/MEK1* p.D67N;
- ATDB102: wild-type, common reference or diluent for all cancer genomic DNA standards.

Quantitative study data would provide values as % mutation and copy numbers for clinically relevant variants, while qualitative data would include the verified presence of thousands of other variants, single nucleotide polymorphism, INDELS and structural variants. It was further outlined that the proposed international standards would be NGS focused as this is currently the only technique available for the parallel analysis of very large numbers of loci. It is known that significant variation exists in platforms, wet lab components and bioinformatics processing – all of which require validation and verification. Nevertheless, the standard materials would also be appropriate for use with other methods such as digital PCR. If successfully endorsed, it was envisaged that the initially proposed WHO international standards would be presented for consideration for establishment by the Committee in 2019.

During discussion, clarification was requested of how the proposed genomic material would perform in comparison with clinical material – commonly, DNA extracted from formalin-fixed paraffin-embedded (FFPE) tissue blocks – and whether there was a need to provide cellular reference materials instead of simply extracted genomic material as proposed. In response it was highlighted that standard development requires the use of homogenous material and this would not be possible if using FFPE. In addition, if cellular material were to be used instead of pre-extracted materials there would still be a large degree of variability in the extraction methods used. Although FFPE is a commonly used approach, it is not the only one currently used by the community, and a common clinical material covering all these methods would not be possible. The proposed genomic material would be suitable for use across multiple methods and should the end user wish to produce a secondary reference material more akin to a clinical sample this would still be possible. Clarity was requested regarding the intention of the group to produce individual members rather than a panel as this meant that the Committee was effectively being asked to endorse a programme of work. It was highlighted in response that such an endorsement had previously been given for the development of VEGF antagonists. In the first instance, it was intended that three WHO international standards would be brought to the Committee for establishment. The Committee endorsed the proposal (WHO/BS/2018.2342) to develop a series of WHO international standards for cancer cell genomes rather than a WHO international reference panel.

7.2.3 Proposed First WHO international standards for *PIK3CA* variants

Phosphatidylinositol-4,5-bisphosphate 3-kinase (PIK3) is a key enzyme in the mTOR signalling pathway involved in cell growth and proliferation, protein translation and synthesis, and apoptosis regulation. Variants of the PIK3 catalytic subunit alpha (*PIK3CA*) gene are the second most frequently mutated cancer gene in all tumours and may lead to persistent activation of the downstream signalling pathway. The variant is associated with poor therapeutic responses in breast, endometrial and colorectal cancers, and with poor patient outcomes in lung cancer. Advances in understanding the effects of *PIK3CA* mutations on therapeutic responses and the development of PIK3-targeted therapies for metastatic breast cancer mean there is now a clear public health need for accurate and sensitive genotyping to ensure correct patient diagnosis, to allow for the use of optimal drug treatments, and to monitor treatment responses and prognosis.

The proposed candidate materials for use as individual international standards would be the four most common tumour-associated *PIK3CA* variants – p.H1047R, p.E545K, p.E542K and p.H1047L (cancer cell lines) – and a wild-type *PIK3CA* (lymphoblastoid cell line). These four variants account for ~66% of all cases of *PIK3CA*-associated cancers. Approximately 5000 lyophilized ampoules of each candidate material would be prepared for evaluation in a range of current methodologies (pyrosequencing, HRM analysis, QPCR, Sanger sequencing and NGS). The primary source of the material would be genomic DNA as this is available in sufficient quantities, and is stable, homogeneous and readily replaceable. Conversely, primary patient material would be hard to obtain and of variable quality. It was envisaged that the four candidate materials initially developed would become individual WHO international standards, with additional variants produced as and when considered necessary. It was anticipated that the first four candidate materials would be presented to the Committee for its consideration in 2022.

The Committee endorsed the proposal (WHO/BS/2018.2342) to develop the First WHO international standards for *PIK3CA* variants.

7.2.4 Proposed Second WHO International Standard for insulin-like growth factor-I (human, recombinant)

Insulin-like growth factor-I (IGF-I) is the principal mediator of the effects of growth hormone, and is the preferred marker for the diagnosis of growth-related disorders. Serum IGF-I levels are usually measured using immunoassays. The First WHO International Standard for IGF-I (human, recombinant) for immunoassays was established in 2008 and is used by manufacturers, and by clinical, academic and doping laboratories to calibrate in-house immunoassay standards. At the current rate of dispatch of 150–200 ampoules per year, stocks of the current WHO international standard are expected to be exhausted in 2020, and a replacement is required to ensure the continued availability of an international standard.

Efforts to obtain recombinant (*E. coli*) human IGF-I from a therapeutic product manufacturer are ongoing, and involve essentially the same source material that was used to produce the current international standard. The new standard will be value-assigned via high-performance liquid chromatography (HPLC) against a primary calibrant and its suitability confirmed using immunoassays. Commutability will also be evaluated. Although primary calibrant vials remain from the international collaborative study conducted to establish the current international standard, the purity profile of the recombinant human IGF-I used is likely to have changed over the last 20 years. This may necessitate the production and value-assignment of a new primary calibrant. To address this, the similarity of the newly donated material and the existing primary calibrant will be evaluated by HPLC before proceeding. It is intended that the source material will be obtained by the end of 2018 with further development work (up to and including definitive fill and post-fill characterization) completed during 2019. An international collaborative study would then be conducted with submission of its outcomes to the Committee in 2020.

During discussion, clarification was requested of the reason for assigning mass units to this standard rather than functional units. It was clarified that clinically, IGF-I is measured in mass units and comparability to clinical practice should be maintained, as had been the case for the first international standard. It was also further clarified that although the purity of the original primary calibrant may have changed, possibly due to denaturation, its specific activity can still be characterized by protein sequencing and HPLC.

The Committee endorsed the proposal (WHO/BS/2018.2342) to develop a Second WHO International Standard for insulin-like growth factor-1 (human, recombinant).

7.2.5 Proposed WHO international standards for enterovirus RNA for NAT-based assays

As the eradication of poliovirus draws near, increased attention is now being given to the diagnosis and treatment of non-polio enteroviruses (EVs). EVs are a common cause of self-limiting febrile illnesses in infants and young children, and the most common cause of meningitis – with infection with some EV types also linked to acute flaccid myelitis and acute flaccid paralysis. Certain EV types, notably EV-A71 and EV-D68, have also been associated with disease outbreaks that occasionally result in significant morbidity and mortality. For example, EV-A71 has been responsible for large outbreaks of hand, foot and mouth disease, while EV-D68 has been associated with severe respiratory disease, occasionally leading to acute flaccid myelitis, in North America and Europe.

Numerous multiplex diagnostic assays that target the highly conserved 5′ untranslated region are now being introduced for the detection of EVs. However, external quality assessment studies have indicated that the sensitivity of such assays varies greatly. There is therefore a need to develop reference materials for the commonly targeted EV-A71, EV-ED68 and Coxsackieviruses

WHO Technical Report Series, No. 1016, 2019

A and B. Given anticipated difficulties in the sourcing of clinical materials it is proposed that candidate materials for use as WHO international standards will be produced collaboratively. It is intended that source materials will be secured by mid-2019.

During discussion, clarification was requested of whether the project would aim to develop a panel of materials or individual international standards for each material. Given the absence of known cross-reactivity in these viruses, it was agreed that individual standards should be developed.

The Committee endorsed the proposal (WHO/BS/2018.2342) to develop WHO international standards for enterovirus RNA for NAT-based assays.

7.2.6 Proposed Fourth WHO International Standard for ferritin (human, recombinant)

The Committee was informed that due to worldwide demand stocks of the current Third WHO International Standard for ferritin (human, recombinant) were now nearing exhaustion. Each year, 200–300 ampoules of this international standard are distributed to clinical laboratories and manufacturers of assay kits. The international standard is used to ensure the comparability of human serum ferritin immunoassay test results across laboratories. To ensure continuity of supply, a replacement international standard was now needed.

To develop candidate material for use as a replacement standard it was intended that human ferritin light chain would be expressed in *E. coli* and diluted in human serum. One acknowledged issue raised by this proposal was the potential difficulty of proving that the recombinant ferritin light chain produced was immunologically similar to that used in the existing standard – since it is diluted in human serum, performing the required western blot assay is complicated. This issue had been addressed at a number of previous meetings, with results to date indicating that a pilot batch of recombinant ferritin exhibited responses parallel to the current standard, with a slight loss of activity due to lyophilization. It is intended that source material will be obtained by the end of 2018. This will be followed by trial fills and external validation by the first half of 2019 and definitive fill and post-fill characterization by the end of 2019. A collaborative study would then be conducted in 2020 with submission of its outcomes to the Committee in 2021.

During discussion, it was pointed out that the recombinant construct for the proposed new standard was not identical to the construct used in the current standard, but was a newly constructed plasmid in a different expression system. However, the genetic sequence was identical to that of the previous construct.

The Committee endorsed the proposal (WHO/BS/2018.2342) to develop a Fourth WHO International Standard for ferritin (human, recombinant).

7.2.7 Proposed First WHO International Reference Panel for microsatellite instability

Microsatellites are short DNA sequences (1–6 base pairs) tandemly repeated throughout the human genome, and are known to be prone to DNA replication error. Microsatellite instability (MSI) is the condition of genetic hypermutability resulting from impaired DNA mismatch repair. Many cancers, particularly colorectal cancer are the result of MSI, the testing for which is routine in the clinical management of colorectal cancer. A status of MSI-high (MSI-H) may be prognostic for improved survival. Immunotherapeutic mAbs that bind to inhibitory PD-1 receptors on T-cells, thus counteracting functional exhaustion, are now becoming available, with one drug now approved for the treatment of any MSI-H solid tumour.

Although MSI testing is traditionally performed by PCR using paired healthy and tumour tissue samples, NGS is a rapidly emerging diagnostic tool. There are challenges in quantifying changes in microsatellite sizings, with a strong reliance on software or manual interpretation. Recent advances in linking immunity, cancer genomics and therapeutics will likely lead to new standards of patient care and substantially increase demand for MSI analysis. Standards are therefore required to help ensure accurate and sensitive diagnostic testing, which will be crucial in selecting patients for immunotherapy.

It is intended that genomic DNA will be prepared from MSI-H and MSI-negative cell lines, ideally using CRISPR engineering. However it was noted that a licence to use CRISPR was required and this issue was still to be resolved. In the event of CRISPR not being available, potential alternative methods would include the use of Lynch syndrome patient lymphoblastoid cell lines or other cancer cell lines widely reported to be MSI-H. Provisional estimates indicate that the timescale for inducing microsatellite sizing changes will be around 2–3 months, with ~5000 ampoules of each material planned for production. It was envisaged that the proposal to establish the reference panel would be submitted to the Committee in 2020 or 2021.

It was clarified during discussion that no technical difficulties were expected in relation to the use of CRISPR. The more likely issues would concern licensure and potentially prohibitive costs. Concerns were expressed regarding the ability of CRISPR technology to generate a stable phenotype – an issue also of potential relevance in the expansion of cell lines. However, it was clarified that in this case it is only the genotype that is important, and this can be controlled and ensured. In addition, a single-culture system approach would be used to provide well-characterized stock materials and control the suitability of cell lines. Discussion also took place on the consensus definition of MSI-H. Currently, five microsatellite markers are assessed and if two or more were high then the material was considered to be MSI-H. However, the use of NGS will mean the assessment of thousands of loci and there would be a need to understand the clinical relevance of the data generated. It was confirmed that NGS technology would be used in the collaborative study to assess the candidate materials. A decision would be taken on whether to create dilutions of different levels of MSI-H or a straight forward MSI-H, MSI-low and MSI-negative panel. It was noted in closing that immunotherapy was a rapidly advancing field and that standardization efforts would need to keep pace.

The Committee endorsed the proposal (WHO/BS/2018.2342) to develop a First WHO International Reference Panel for microsatellite instability.

7.2.8 Proposed First WHO International Standard for *Mycobacterium tuberculosis* DNA for NAT-based assays

Tuberculosis (TB) is a major public health concern, especially in LMIC where diagnostic facilities are inadequate. Moving towards the ambitious target of the international health community to end TB worldwide will require the development of more accurate and rapid diagnostic tests for TB. Until recently, the diagnosis of TB has been based mainly on sputum-smear microscopy or culture techniques. Although, these methods are effective in diagnosing highly infectious TB they are less effective for the early diagnosis of individuals with less-pronounced symptoms. In addition, these methods require long turnaround times. More sensitive and rapid diagnostic tests based on the molecular detection (nucleic acid amplification) of the DNA of *Mycobacterium tuberculosis* are now available, with many more in development – including point-of-care tests. In combination with systems for centralized testing, the resulting faster turnaround of test results will allow for the more rapid initiation of treatment.

At a WHO workshop held in 2018 to discuss advances in TB diagnostic technologies and the associated need for suitable standards for molecular detection, it was proposed that a candidate reference material be produced from inactivated laboratory strain H37Rv. It was further proposed that this material could be lyophilized at a concentration of ~10^6 genome copies per ml in a universal buffer, with DNA extraction performed in sputum provided as a matrix for testing. Ideally, a TB diagnostic test should also include drug-susceptibility testing to allow for the screening of resistance mutations. In addition to the single reference material, it would therefore be necessary to subsequently develop a reference panel comprising strains with different resistance mutations.

A possible source of H37Rv had now been identified and further expert discussions held on the potential limitations of using sputum as a matrix. In addition, concerns had been raised in relation to the inactivation and lyophilization processes to be used, and the effects these may have on the quantification of DNA in the preparation. In advance of a collaborative study to establish a reference material for *M. tuberculosis* a pilot study would therefore be conducted to compare different inactivation methods and to evaluate the use of frozen versus freeze-dried materials. As mycobacteria suspensions tend to clump (thus affecting the quantification of DNA), attention will also be given to ensuring the homogeneity of filling in large-scale production. It is intended that source material will be obtained in early 2019 with trial fills, definitive fill and post-fill characterization completed by late 2019. A collaborative study would then be conducted with submission of its outcomes to the Committee in 2020.

During discussion, it was confirmed that the candidate material would be inactivated. Inputs were also received regarding recent experience in the use of artificial sputum, and an offer made to share existing formulations for use in the proposed study.

The Committee endorsed the proposal (WHO/BS/2018.2342) to develop a First WHO International Standard for *Mycobacterium tuberculosis* DNA for NAT-based assays and a subsequent panel containing resistant mutations.

7.2.9 Proposed First WHO International Standard for anti-thyroid peroxidase antibodies

The NIBSC reference reagent for anti-thyroid microsome serum (NIBSC code 66/387) was produced in the 1960s from a pool of serum from three patients who exhibited autoimmune anti-thyroid microsome activity. The target of this anti-thyroid microsome autoimmunity had since been identified as thyroid peroxidase (TPO). The development of immunoassays to detect anti-TPO autoantibodies for the diagnosis of thyroid autoimmune diseases (for example, Hashimoto's thyroiditis) and of hypo- and hyperthyroidism led to the worldwide adoption of reference reagent 66/387 for their calibration. Stocks of this reagent are now depleted and given its widespread adoption there is an urgent need to develop a replacement standard.

The replacement strategy proposed is to replace the current reference reagent with a First WHO International Standard for anti-thyroid peroxidase antibodies. Serum, source plasma or recovered plasma from high titre anti-TPO donors will be purchased (or donated) and then pooled to provide bulk material for the production of a candidate material. The candidate material will be assessed and value assigned by comparison with the current reference reagent by immunoassay in a collaborative study. Given an average level of demand for the current reference reagent of 125 ampoules per year over the last three years, it is estimated that 2000–2500 ampoules of the replacement international standard would be sufficient for 15–20 years.

Issues raised by the proposal include the possible need for additional development work to ensure continuity between the unitage of the current reference reagent and the assigned IU value of the candidate material. In addition, as the epitope coverage of 66/387 is unknown there may be differences in this regard in the replacement and future materials. However, the likelihood of this is considered to be low as the majority of antibodies arise from only two major epitopes, with the majority being of one antibody class (IgG). It is intended that source material will be obtained in late 2018 with trial fills, definitive fill and post-fill characterization completed by the end of 2019. A collaborative study would then be conducted in 2020 with submission of its outcomes to the Committee in 2021.

During discussion, it was clarified that in the case of the current reference reagent the antibody content is measured in quantitative units. If continuity between these units and the proposed IU of the replacement standard cannot be achieved then this might result in some early issues in the field but this should not prevent the establishment of the international standard.

The Committee endorsed the proposal (WHO/BS/2018.2342) to develop a First WHO International Standard for anti-thyroid peroxidase antibodies.

7.2.10 Proposed extension of the First WHO International Reference Panel for HIV-1 circulating recombinant forms RNA for NAT-based assays

HIV-1 is a highly diverse virus with many known subtypes and variants. In 2001, an HIV-1 RNA panel for use in NAT-based assays was developed to cover the "main" subtypes. In 2013, an HIV-1 CRF panel was developed comprising 10 commonly identified CRFs. However, due to random recombination events during replication, the evolution of HIV-1 variants continues. It was therefore proposed that a further 6–8 samples of currently circulating variants be developed and assessed, either for addition to the current CRF panel or for use in developing a new standalone panel. The project would be a collaborative effort with CBER assuming responsibility for sourcing the CRFs and for producing high-titre inactivated candidate materials. These materials would then be passed to NIBSC for lyophilization and distribution for a collaborative study in which CBER would also be participants. It is intended that source material will be obtained in 2019, with definitive fill and post-fill characterization completed by the end of 2019. A collaborative study would then be conducted with submission of its outcomes to the Committee in 2020.

The Committee agreed that this project would provide up-to-date complementary materials for use in the current HIV-1 CRF RNA panel. Extensive discussion then took place around the final naming of such a panel and whether this would be an expansion of the current panel or a standalone resource. In either case, care would be needed in the nomenclature used to describe these panels to ensure clarity in the user community. The Committee agreed that the best approach might be to develop a standalone panel and discussion centred on dispensing with the traditional nomenclature of "First", "Second" etc. as this would imply replacement which was not the case. The suggestion was made to instead use the year of establishment in the panel title. As this approach had not been used before, it was felt this would require further discussion.

The Committee endorsed the proposal (WHO/BS/2018.2342) to extend the First WHO International Reference Panel for HIV-1 circulating recombinant forms RNA for NAT-based assays on the understanding that the issue of nomenclature for the establishment of additional international reference reagents requires resolution.

7.2.11 Proposed First WHO international standards for circulating tumour DNA

Cancer patients often have significantly higher levels of circulating cell-free DNA (cfDNA) than healthy individuals and this is now considered to be a significant diagnostic marker. The use of liquid biopsies rather than standard biopsies is increasing due to their rapid turnaround time and minimally invasive nature. The analysis of tumour cells and tumour-derived products in the blood, including circulating cell-free tumour DNA (ctDNA), relies on the detection of chromatin fragments. An increasing number of ctDNA tests were now becoming available using both PCR and NGS technologies. However, concerns have recently been expressed regarding the use of ctDNA tests, particularly in light of insufficient evidence of their clinical validity and utility for majority of ctDNA assays, and apparent discordance between ctDNA and solid tumour results. Clearly, the provision of suitable reference materials would help to address these concerns.

It was therefore proposed that four materials would be developed covering the four most clinically relevant EGFR variants – namely, exon 19 deletion(s), T790M, L858R and wild-type EGFR. Each candidate material would comprise pooled commercial human plasma spiked with synthetic DNA oligonucleotides and/or chromatin fragments from (CRISPR-engineered) cell lines. Diluting the ctDNA standards with wild-type cfDNA-containing plasma would produce standards across a range of mutation levels prior to provision to the participants of a planned collaborative study. Around 5000 lyophilized ampoules of each of the freeze-dried candidate materials would be developed. It was acknowledged that it will not be possible to produce standards for all clinically relevant variants in the first instance, but that further standards could be developed over time. It was expected that the candidate materials would be suitable for the derivation of secondary standards for use in QPCR, NGS and droplet digital PCR methodologies, and for the calibration of commercial assays and kits.

Source materials (plasma, oligonucleotides and cell lines) had now been obtained and a pilot study completed. Further studies were planned starting in

2018 with definitive fill and post-fill characterization expected to be completed in 2020. A collaborative study would then be conducted with submission of its outcomes to the Committee in 2021.

It was highlighted during discussion that ctDNA was often present in very low levels, thus raising issues for its assured detection – an issue that would not necessarily be addressed if the dilution of materials was left to the end user. In response, it was pointed out that pilot studies were being conducted to better understand low-level assay detection using the materials that will be provided. A second pilot study was also planned involving collaborators developing NGS for detecting low-percentage mutations in liquid biopsies. The outcome of these studies would help determine if the end user would perform the serial dilutions. It was also clarified that the material to be provided in the study would be fragmented so as to be representative of clinical samples.

The Committee endorsed the proposal (WHO/BS/2018.2342) to develop First WHO international standards for circulating tumour DNA.

7.2.12 Proposed First WHO Reference Reagent for *Babesia microti* DNA for NAT-based assays

Babesia microti is a parasitic protozoan which infects erythrocytes causing a malaria-like illness known as babesiosis. The highest prevalence of babesiosis occurs in the USA and is a combination of natural infections and transfusion-transmitted infections. Although a variety of *Babesia* species exist, *B. microti* is the most common cause of infections. In 2018, two screening tests for *B. microti* were licensed in the USA. Evidence indicates that NAT-based assays are highly effective in identifying low-grade early infections and chronic asymptomatic infections in prospective blood donors. However, due to the intraerythrocytic nature of B. microti and the presence of potentially low-grade infections such assays need to be of the highest sensitivity. There is therefore a clear need for the provision of reference materials to enable manufactures to develop competitive and sensitive tests.

It is intended that a candidate standard for *B. microti* genetic material is obtained from blood-stage parasites grown in DBA/2 mice. The genetic material will be characterized using the nucleotide sequencing of at least five parasite genes and will be quantified by PCR. Candidate material will be lyophilized for use in an international collaborative study alongside human blood spiked with known counts of *B. microti* and murine red blood cells infected with *B. microti*. It was acknowledged that finding laboratories outside the USA that are routinely testing for B. microti may be challenging.

The Committee endorsed the proposal (WHO/BS/2018.2342) to develop a First WHO Reference Reagent for *Babesia microti* DNA for NAT-based assays.

7.2.13 Update on the development of WHO international reference preparations for *Plasmodium vivax*

The WHO 5-year Strategic Plan (2019–2023) (see section 2.1.1) was developed to adapt the regulatory support activities of WHO to country needs and has been used as the basis of discussions with donors funding WHO work in this area. A recent successful application had been made for Global Fund support in the development of WHO quality standards in priority areas that are congruent with the Global Funds' strategic priorities. Following consultation with the WHO prequalification of IVDs programme and WHOCCs to gain insight into the areas of greatest need, it was agreed that funding would be provided for the development of WHO international standards for antigens of *Plasmodium vivax* used for the potency control of diagnostic test kits.

An overview of recent standardization efforts for *P. vivax* was therefore provided to the Committee. In October 2017, the Committee had endorsed projects to develop WHO international standards for *P. vivax* antigens and a WHO international reference reagent for use in *P. vivax* serology. In the case of the antigen project, candidate materials will be derived from a pool of clinical *P. vivax* samples with a focus placed on lactate dehydrogenase as this is the only antigen currently detected by a significant number of rapid diagnostic tests for *P. vivax*. Clinical material had now been sourced from Peru and trial lyophilization was in progress. It was envisaged that the results of a collaborative study would be submitted to the Committee in 2020. In addition, acute serology samples were also available from the same clinical material, with convalescent serology samples also having been obtained from the Singapore blood bank. This would likely be sufficient for the generation of the serological reference materials but efforts to obtain clinical samples from India were also ongoing. The submission of study results to the Committee was also planned for 2020.

In addition to the need for international standards and reference reagents, there is also an urgent need for external quality control materials for assay monitoring and validation. As in vitro culturing is not possible for *P. vivax*, one sustainable approach to the provision of antigenic run-control materials is the use of recombinant proteins. There are however concerns regarding the use of such materials, and it was noted in the previous *P. falciparum* study that recombinant proteins did not perform as suitably as whole parasite material, raising questions over their commutability. An alternative approach was therefore outlined involving the use of allelic replacement of *P. vivax* lactate dehydrogenase in either *P. falciparum* or *P. knowlesi*. *P. knowlesi* is thought to be a closer match to *P. vivax* and CRISPR would be available in both cases. Following such manipulation, the culture-derived materials could be formulated and assessed as had been the case for *P. falciparum*. If such materials were produced in time, they could be jointly assessed in the international standards study.

During discussion it was pointed out that the ultimate goal of the Global Fund was to make products available to market and it was important to be mindful of the link between this and standards development. It was also suggested that if the use of recombinant antigens proved to be successful then clones could be used in assay development which in turn may assist in the timely reintroduction of blood donors into the donation system. In view of the short time frames involved in these particular projects, the Committee was asked to consider giving its general endorsement on the understanding that consultations were still ongoing. After due consideration, the Committee agreed and indicated its general endorsement of the proposals made.

8. International reference materials – standards for use in public health emergencies

All reference materials established at the meeting are listed in Annex 5.

 ## WHO International Standards and Reference Reagents – standards for use in public health emergencies

 ### First WHO International Standard for anti-Asian lineage Zika virus antibody (human)

More than 86 countries have now reported evidence of Zika infections with two main lineages identified – African and Asian. Following several outbreaks in the last 11 years, there has been an expansion in the range of assays now available for Zika virus detection. These have included NAT-based assays designated by WHO under its EUAL procedure and those approved through FDA Emergency Use Authorization. In addition, 45 vaccines were currently in development with several of these now undergoing Phase I or Phase II clinical trials.

An international collaborative study had been undertaken to evaluate preparations of sera and plasma obtained from individuals infected with Zika virus, along with purified immunoglobulins derived from trans-chromosomal bovines immunized with Zika virus immunogens for their suitability to serve as the First WHO International Standard for anti-Asian lineage Zika virus antibody (human). It was envisaged that such a standard could be utilized in diagnosis, vaccine evaluation and serosurveillance. A range of antibody sample preparations were tested along with additional negative antibody samples and dengue virus serotype-specific samples in a blinded manner using anti-ZIKV assays established in the participant laboratories. A total of 28 datasets were returned by 19 laboratories in six countries. Assays types used included qualitative anti-Zika IgM ELISA (n = 6), qualitative anti-Zika IgG assays (n = 3) quantitative anti-IgG ELISA (n = 3) and neutralization assays (n = 14).

Study results indicated that all the human serum/plasma samples were relatively concordant in the assays used. Analysed data showed a reduction in inter-laboratory variation when values were expressed relative to the candidate sample (NIBSC code 16/352). Although all convalescent plasma/serum samples were positive for anti-ZIKV IgM, their potency could not be quantified as the IgM assays performed were qualitative only. The candidate material 16/352 – a clinical pool of convalescent sera – was selected as the proposed international standard. As this material had also been aliquoted into a relatively large number of ampoules (~2000) a longer period would elapse before a replacement was needed.

The specificity of anti-Zika virus antibodies in the candidate preparation was addressed by the inclusion of the anti-dengue virus reference reagents with the majority of assays exhibiting no cross-reactivity. Such cross-reactivity was mainly observed in neutralization assays, where the target protein is known to have a common epitope with other flaviviruses, mainly dengue viruses. It was therefore proposed that the candidate material 16/352 be established as the First WHO International Standard for anti-Asian lineage Zika virus antibody (human) with an arbitrary assigned unitage of 1000 IU/ml, corresponding to 250 IU/ampoule.

Clarification was requested regarding the suitable application of this reference material. It was confirmed that it would only be suitable for use in Asian-lineage Zika virus neutralization assays and that this would be made clear in the IFU. Due to the limited amount of study data generated on African-lineage Zika virus neutralization assays and on the use of ELISA, a definitive conclusion on the suitability of the international standard for these purposes cannot yet be made. This topic may become the subject of further investigations. Discussion then turned to the potential use of the material in understanding the cross-reactivity of other flaviviruses. Given the common neutralizing epitopes shared by Zika and dengue viruses the inability to obtain human material that did not give a positive signal for dengue was unsurprising. Further work on this will take place as part of the project endorsed by the Committee in 2017 to replace the current First WHO reference reagents for dengue virus subtypes 1–4. The Committee considered the report of the study (WHO/BS/2018.2345) and recommended that the candidate material 16/352 be established as the First WHO International Standard for anti-Asian lineage Zika virus antibody (human) with an arbitrary assigned unitage of 250 IU/ampoule.

8.2 Proposed new projects and updates – standards for use in public health emergencies

8.2.1 Proposed First WHO International Reference Reagent for MERS-CoV

The Committee was reminded that in 2012 WHO had initiated a project to evaluate the comparability of various commercial and in-house serological assays developed following the emergence of the Middle East respiratory syndrome coronavirus (MERS-CoV). A panel of both positive and negative materials had been developed consisting of both clinically derived convalescent sera and synthetic IgG generated using a humanized trans-chromosomal bovine model. The materials were then assessed across a range of serological assays, including neutralization assays (both wild-type virus and pseudovirus assays), ELISA (including both in-house and commercial assays for S protein and N protein), immunofluorescence assays and microarray assays. Ten laboratories in a number of global regions participated, with a total of 27 datasets being returned.

Results highlighted that in a number of cases the assays were in good agreement. However, many assays could not detect a low-positive pooled human sera sample. This sample could only be correctly identified as positive in one assay and was below the limit of detection in all others. The sample comprised a pool of six sera all from laboratory-confirmed cases of MERS-CoV. In addition to understanding assay performance, additional data analysis was conducted to determine the extent to which the trans-chromosomal material included in the study also displayed a harmonizing effect on the results obtained for the positive samples. Although the largest harmonization effect was exhibited by pooled human sera from confirmed cases, it was apparent that use of the bovine trans-chromosomal sample raised against whole virus resulted in a large improvement compared with the raw mean estimates. Unfortunately, one assay type assessed in the study failed to detect this material.

As the samples evaluated in the study were only available in small volumes, no material remained from which to produce a reference preparation. In order to move forward and evaluate a candidate material that could be established as a WHO reference preparation for MERS-CoV new materials would now need to be sourced and evaluated in a collaborative study. It was highlighted that continual efforts had been made during the 6-year duration of the project to source further donations of confirmed MERS-CoV-positive patent sera but to no avail. The question therefore arose of whether it would be better to wait for donation of a positive patient sera or pool as this would seem to be the most suitable material for developing the proposed international standard or to proceed immediately with the evaluation of the trans-chromosomal bovine material raised against whole virus. This latter approach would allow for the more timely development of a reference reagent that would still provide significant benefit to a large number of users.

The Committee noted the comprehensive update provided and appreciated the difficulties involved in sourcing clinical materials. Clarification was also sought of the likely causes of the single assay type failing to detect the trans-chromosomal material, and the possibility was raised that this may have been an artefact of the material, the assay or the laboratory performing it. As the assay had only been used by one laboratory in the study, this was not immediately clear. During any wider study it was suggested that this assay type should, if possible, be included and assessed by more than one laboratory. The Committee felt that there would be no benefit in delaying the development of a suitable reference preparation and that larger volumes of the bovine trans-chromosomal material raised against whole virus should be obtained and assessed in a full international collaborative study. If found to be suitable the material could be established as a WHO international reference reagent with a unit value. If suitable clinical material was subsequently sourced this could then become the WHO international standard with a value assigned in IU. The Committee therefore endorsed the proposal to develop a First WHO International Reference Reagent for MERS-CoV.

8.2.2 Proposed WHO international standards for emerging and re-emerging viruses with epidemic potential

The Committee was reminded that as part of the global effort to better respond to future epidemics WHO had developed its R&D Blueprint. A list of priority pathogens had been developed which included Crimean-Congo haemorrhagic fever (CCHF) virus, filoviruses (Ebola virus and Marburg virus), Lassa virus, highly pathogenic emerging coronaviruses relevant to humans (MERS-CoV and severe acute respiratory syndrome), Nipah virus, Rift Valley fever virus and Zika virus. A brief outline was then provided for all of the priority pathogens for which the development of WHO international standards was being proposed. The Committee was informed that no vaccine or treatment was currently available for any of the diseases under discussion – each of which had a high case-fatality rate. Materials for developing antibody standards would be sourced from a pool of plasma/serum from convalescent individuals, from vaccinees or from immunized trans-chromosomal bovines. Sourcing material from endemic regions had been identified as a challenge and setting up the required material transfer agreements and governmental approvals may take time.

A number of biosafety and biosecurity issues would also need to be addressed as all the viruses in question are BSL4 agents and are listed in the UK Terrorism Act 2006. Previously approved standard operating procedures for the reception and handling of Ebola virus antibody material will be followed for other BSL4 viruses. In the case of RNA standards, the UK Terrorism Act 2006 again raises issues for the production and distribution of standards based on inactivated viruses. Alternatively, viral RNA could be packaged inside lentiviral particles, as was the approach used for developing the First WHO international reference reagents for Ebola virus RNA for NAT-based assays. Such a reagent could be developed quickly and would be safe and non-infectious. However, at present insufficient commutability studies had been conducted with such constructs to prove their comparability with the actual virus.

Other entities working to address needs and gaps in the development of relevant vaccines include the UK Vaccine Network and the Coalition for Epidemic Preparedness Innovations (CEPI). A CEPI biological standards and assays working group had now been established to bring together stakeholders in the development of biological standards, assays and animal models essential for vaccine characterization and evaluation relevant to the WHO R&D Blueprint and CEPI prioritized targets. Task forces for the development of vaccine and IVD standards for Lassa virus, Nipah virus and MERS-CoV had been established or were in the process of being established. WHO would remain closely involved with these and related developments to ensure consistency with the WHO mission to establish international standards for use in PHEs. In addition, NIBSC had developed a strategic plan for developing new reference materials in this area, and was currently prioritizing the development of international antibody and RNA standards for Lassa virus, Nipah virus, CCHF virus, and Marburg and Sudan viruses. These are intended for use in the standardization of serological assays and/or potency testing of antibodies. Intended users would include clinical and public health laboratories, vaccine and therapeutic antibody manufacturers, assay kit manufacturers and research laboratories. Similar work on Zika virus and chikungunya virus had already been completed and work was in progress on MERS-CoV.

During discussion, it was noted that the establishment of WHO international reference preparations by the Committee might be facilitated by the work of CEPI in collecting convalescent material for Lassa fever, and subsequently for Nipah virus infection. Other governmental and academic avenues were being explored for obtaining source materials for CCHF and Sudan virus. No progress had yet being made in sourcing materials for Marburg virus infections. It was envisaged that the first candidate standards to be submitted to the Committee for its consideration would be for Lassa virus, Nipah virus and CCHF, with a projected submission date of 2020.

The issue of specific considerations applying to each of the individual standards to be developed was raised. These include the need to consider genetic variability and other potential variables and may necessitate the production of reference panels rather than a single reference material. It was also highlighted that while such considerations are important, the need for the timely development of standards does not always allow for the use of materials considered to be ideal. Given previous incidents in which the response of the international health community had been perceived to be slow, there may be a need to consider the use of non-ideal materials, particularly in situations in which the most suitable clinical materials were not immediately available.

WHO as a recognized global organization had an important role to play in facilitating the sharing of clinical materials across national borders during outbreaks. The work of the WHO Office of the Legal Counsel in addressing legal issues during clinical trials might also be relevant to the country-to-country transfer of clinical materials. It was acknowledged that many of the priority agents required containment at BSL4 and needed to meet specific country requirements for their handling. It was proposed that WHO compile a list of BSL4 containment laboratories detailing their location and any in-country restrictions on the handling of specific pathogens, and then share this list with WHOCCs.

The Committee emphasized the need for effective communication between WHO, CEPI, technical drafting groups, WHOCCs and other entities in order to ensure the coordination of efforts now being made to develop WHO international reference preparations for use in PHEs. The precise roles and responsibilities of all the different organizations should be clearly defined and better coordinated. Improved sharing of information between the stakeholders was also urged and the suggestion was made that WHO might consider facilitating a forum for exchanging information if none currently existed.

Following further discussion and clarification of timelines, funding and details of the proposed collaborative studies, as well as of issues related to the donation of reference materials, the Committee endorsed the proposals set out in WHO/BS/2018.2342 to develop WHO international standards for the indicated priority pathogens.

9. International reference materials –
vaccines and related substances

9.1 WHO International Standards and Reference Reagents – vaccines and related substances

9.1.1 Second WHO International Reference Cell Bank of MRC-5 cells

The original seed stock of Medical Research Council cell strain 5 (MRC-5) cells was established in the 1960s in the United Kingdom and cells from this original stock were used for decades in the development and production of a number of major viral vaccines. In 2007, a replacement MRC-5 cell bank became the WHO reference cell bank (RCB). The Committee was reminded that the purpose of WHO RCBs was to provide a well-characterized cell seed material for the generation of an MCB by manufacturers, with the expectation that the material complies with WHO guidance.

The Committee was reminded that the replacement MRC-5 cell bank had been developed at a slightly higher passage level than the original stock. Unfortunately, issues concerning low cell numbers per vial and even higher than reported passage level had resulted in its withdrawal. A decision had then been made to create a second replacement RCB of MRC-5 cells. In 2014, 189 vials of the proposed replacement standard at $\sim 4.3 \times 10^6$ cells/vial and a population doubling level of 13 was produced and fully characterized (bank number: 660902-M02). A full master file had been produced which included information on the history and production of the original cell bank, and extensive information on the production, storage and testing history of the proposed replacement RCB.

It was pointed out that establishing this material as the Second WHO International Reference Cell Bank of MRC-5 cells would allow for WHO oversight. It was further proposed that a procedure similar to that used for WHO Vero RCB 10-87 be used to review and approve requests for the material. At the current rate of distribution it was envisaged that 660902-M02 would last for around 16 years.

The Committee considered the report of the study (WHO/BS/2018.2347) and recommended that the MRC-5 cell bank 660902-M02 be established as the Second WHO International Reference Cell Bank of MRC-5 cells. It further recommended that a procedure for reviewing and approving requests for this material be developed by WHO and NIBSC based on well-defined criteria.

9.1.2 Seventh WHO International Standard for rabies vaccine

The public health and economic impacts of rabies remain substantial, especially in Asia and Africa. Rabies vaccines for human and veterinary use are produced in many countries and their potency is an important indicator of the consistency of production batches with respect to the level of potency shown to be efficacious in clinical trials. The currently required potency test for rabies vaccine for human use is the National Institutes of Health (NIH) mouse potency test. This assay is also used to test product stability for the purpose of establishing shelf-life. In both cases, minimum potency requirements are expressed in IU.

The surface glycoprotein of the rabies virus is the immunogenic antigen in rabies vaccines responsible for conferring protection. Quantification of this surface glycoprotein in rabies vaccines – for example, using SRD or ELISA – is routinely performed during vaccine manufacture, particularly at the final bulk stage to determine the final antigen content per dose of vaccine. In light of this and of the 3Rs approach to animal testing, EDQM and other organizations are developing an ELISA method using mAbs against the trimeric form of the glycoprotein to replace the NIH test for determining rabies vaccine potency.

The WHO International Standard for rabies vaccine is used by manufacturers of human and veterinary vaccines, and by control-testing laboratories, for the standardization of potency and glycoprotein assays. The Committee was informed that stocks of the current WHO international standard were essentially depleted, and that a candidate replacement international standard (NIBSC code 16/204) had been obtained. This material had been prepared from a purified and inactivated bulk of Vero cell-derived Pitman Moore strain rabies vaccine using the same process used to prepare the current international standard and donated by the same manufacturer.

An international collaborative study had been conducted in 2017/18 to assess the suitability of the candidate material 16/204 to serve as the Seventh WHO International Standard for rabies vaccine. The aim of the study was to assess the candidate material against the current international standard in the NIH mouse potency assay as well as in the in vitro assays of rabies vaccines for glycoprotein content. Sixteen laboratories from 12 countries assayed the candidate standard (in duplicate) with 10 datasets returned for the NIH mouse potency test, nine for the ELISA and six for the SRD assays. The overall geometric mean potency of the candidate material was 8.9 IU/ampoule in NIH tests. The mean rabies glycoprotein antigen content of the candidate material using in vitro assays was 2.45 IU/ampoule in ELISA and 2.9 IU/ampoule in SRD. Inter-laboratory GCV for the candidate material 16/204 was 51% in NIH tests, and 10.5% and 8.2% in ELISA and SRD assays respectively. These results indicate that the performance of the candidate material was comparable to that of the current international standard during its establishment. Stability data obtained over 12 months indicated an initial drop of 3.8% in glycoprotein content for ampoules stored at −20 °C compared to those stored at −70 °C, with no additional decrease observed in samples stored at 4 °C and 20 °C. Pending the results of ongoing accelerated degradation studies to predict its stability upon long-term storage and shipment at ambient temperatures, the candidate material would be dispatched on dry ice.

The Committee considered the report of the study (WHO/BS/2018.2335) and recommended that the candidate material 16/204 be established as the Seventh WHO International Standard for rabies vaccine with an assigned unitage of 8.9 IU/ampoule when assayed in the NIH mouse potency test. In addition, for the measurement of glycoprotein content in vitro, the candidate material was established with an assigned unitage of 2.5 IU/ampoule in ELISA and 2.9 IU/ampoule in SRD assays. It was considered that the assignment of IU per ampoule (and not per ml) would help avoid pre-dilution confusion. In addition, the unitage for use in ELISA had been rounded up to 2.5 IU/ampoule following recalculation by EDQM and NIBSC statisticians. The Committee highlighted the need to emphasize in the IFU the importance of using the precise dilution of the standard indicated above for the calibration of each of the three assay types to avoid issues encountered in the use of the previous international standard.

9.1.3 First WHO international standards for meningococcal serogroups W and Y polysaccharides

Invasive meningococcal disease causes mortality and morbidity worldwide, particularly in infants. With the incidence of meningococcal group C (MenC) disease now under control in many countries through the implementation of routine vaccination, the remaining disease burden is largely caused by other serogroups, including MenB, MenW and MenY. Meningococcal polysaccharide conjugate vaccines have now been in use for over 20 years with plain polysaccharide vaccines previously available. The first meningococcal conjugate vaccine only contained polysaccharide from MenC. Subsequently, MenA, MenW and MenY polysaccharides were added to produce tetravalent conjugate formulations, with MenX conjugates now in development. Given the complex and ever-changing epidemiology of the different serogroups across different geographical regions, the most effective means of preventing disease remains vaccination against as many groups as possible.

With several manufacturers now producing polysaccharide or polysaccharide conjugate vaccines there is a continued need to harmonize the measurement of the polysaccharide content of these products. Prior to the introduction of WHO international standards for MenC, MenA and MenX polysaccharides, the standardization of vaccine polysaccharide content measurement was problematic due to the wide variety of methods and standards employed by different manufacturers and control laboratories. The quantification of both total and free (unconjugated) polysaccharide content is crucial in determining vaccine potency and is primarily achieved using physicochemical assays using polysaccharide, sialic acid, glucose or galactose standards. Commonly used assays include the Resorcinol assay for the measurement of sialic acid content, and high-performance anion exchange chromatography with pulsed amperometric detection (HPAEC-PAD).

The Committee was reminded that a proposal to assign unitage to candidate polysaccharide standards for MenW and MenY based on quantitative nuclear magnetic resonance (qNMR) for their use as primary calibrators of secondary in-house standards in physicochemical assays had been endorsed by the Committee in 2015. Two candidate materials for use as MenW and MenY international standards (NIBSC codes 16/152 and 16/206 respectively) had been donated by a manufacturer and assessed for their suitability in an international collaborative study. Twelve laboratories from 11 countries had participated in the study with seven performing qNMR spectroscopy, six performing HPAEC-PAD, six performing the Resorcinol assay and one laboratory each performing HPLC, Anthrone and Nephelometry assays. Following the assignment of unitage to the candidate MenW and MenY polysaccharide candidate materials using qNMR and measurement of the degree of O-acetylation of both polysaccharides, an evaluation was made of the suitability of each candidate standard compared against in-house standards. The mean estimates of polysaccharide content obtained for each of the candidate materials and in-house standards using qNMR, HPAEC-PAD and Resorcinol assays were in good agreement. However, upon analysis, the results of unitage assignment using qNMR exhibited a higher than expected degree of variability without obvious explanation. Given this high degree of variability, it was proposed to the Committee that the unitage assignments should be based instead upon the results obtained using the Resorcinol assay.

The Committee considered the report of the study (WHO/BS/2018.2336) and the information that had been presented. The particularly high degree of variability of quantitation results obtained using the qNMR assay was noted, along with the proposal to assign unitage based on the results of the Resorcinol assay. However, the Committee felt that the study report would need to be significantly updated before it could confidently establish the proposed standards, and that the collaborative study participants would need to agree to the revisions made. The Committee therefore deferred decision on these standards and looked forward to receiving an updated report at its next meeting.

9.1.4 First WHO International Standard for Sabin inactivated poliomyelitis vaccine

The eradication of wild poliovirus type 2 (WPV2) in 2015 was followed in 2016 by the removal of the type 2 component from the live-attenuated OPV. The switch from trivalent OPV (tOPV) containing all three poliovirus serotypes to bivalent OPV (bOPV) was intended to prevent further cases of poliomyelitis caused by circulating vaccine-derived poliovirus type 2. Making this switch required the global introduction of IPV – which is not associated with vaccine-related paralysis – in all routine immunization programmes to maintain immunity levels against type 2 polioviruses. The successful eradication of

WPV2 and near completion of WPV1 and WPV3 eradication also means that laboratory containment of all wild-type polioviruses will soon be required (see section 3.4.3). In the context of such containment, the production of IPV using Sabin live-attenuated strains instead of the wild-type poliovirus is considered to be safer. As demand for IPV is now increasing, numerous manufacturers are producing, or planning to produce, Sabin IPV (sIPV) with licensed products already being used in China and Japan.

The potency of IPV is measured in vitro using a validated ELISA with suitable reference preparations and is expressed in D-Antigen (D-Ag) units in line with the WHO Recommendations to assure the quality, safety and efficacy of poliomyelitis vaccines (inactivated). The current Third WHO International Standard for inactivated poliomyelitis vaccine is used by manufacturers and control laboratories to calibrate laboratory reference reagents. However, the Committee was reminded that a collaborative study had shown that this international standard was not suitable for determining the D-Ag content of sIPV products. In the absence of specific sIPV reference standards and well-defined dose requirements current sIPV products vary greatly. A proposal to develop and evaluate an international standard specifically for sIPV D-Ag had been endorsed by the Committee in 2016.

An international collaborative study involving 13 laboratories in eight counties had now been conducted to evaluate candidate materials for potential establishment as the First WHO International Standard for Sabin inactivated poliomyelitis vaccine. Candidate materials and study samples were donated by manufacturers, with two of the candidate materials (NIBSC codes 17/130 and 17/160) tested for their D-Ag content per ml by ELISA. No significant differences were found between the two materials, which were tested alongside three other sIPV products and two conventional IPV reference samples. Study results confirmed the unsuitability of the current international standard for conventional IPV in standardizing the determination of D-Ag content in sIPV products. A clear improvement was noted in the degree of inter-laboratory agreement observed in ELISA D-Ag measurements of sIPV products when using in-house methods in combination with either of the two candidate homologous sIPV materials as a reference. On the basis of the data obtained, neither of the two candidate materials appeared to offer an advantage over the other. Stability studies demonstrated that both candidate materials were stable at temperatures used for long-term storage (−70 °C) and short-term laboratory manipulation (4–20 °C). However, both materials were found to be less stable during storage at −20 °C, particularly 17/160 for which no D-Ag could be detected after 9 months. There was a loss in potency for candidate 17/130 after long-term storage at 4 °C but not for candidate 17/160 which remained stable over the 9-month analysis period.

It had been concluded that either of candidate materials 17/130 and 17/160, would be suitable to serve as an international standard. However, the candidate material 17/160 showed marginally better overall results in terms of assay validity, intra- and inter-laboratory variability and overall thermal stability profiles. Noting the inconsistencies observed between the antigenic properties of conventional IPV and sIPV, and the need for homologous reference materials to accurately measure the antigen content of these products, the suggestion had been made that a new antigen unit – the Sabin D-Ag Unit (SDU) – should be defined specifically for sIPV and independent of the conventional D-Ag units used for cIPV products. This would prevent confusion when using any new sIPV international standard or future sIPV references calibrated against it, to assign antigen potencies to sIPV products.

The Committee agreed with the proposals set out in the report of the study (WHO/BS/2018.2338) and recommended that the candidate material 17/160 be established as the First WHO International Standard for Sabin inactivated poliomyelitis vaccine with individually assigned unitages of 100 SDU/ml for poliovirus type 1, 100 SDU/ml for poliovirus type 2 and 100 SDU/ml for poliovirus type 3. Since this new international standard had only been validated to measure the SDU content of sIPV using in vitro assays, the Committee agreed to the further proposal that a study be undertaken to evaluate its performance using in vivo rat potency assays. The Committee also recommended that already-licensed sIPV products be recalibrated for SDU content against the new international standard, and that the IFU of the conventional IPV standard be updated to the effect that it was only to be used in the evaluation of conventional IPV products.

9.2 Proposed new projects and updates – vaccines and related substances

9.2.1 Update on the development of influenza virus pathogenicity standards

As requested by the Committee in 2017, an update was provided on the progress made towards the development of influenza virus pathogenicity standards. The Committee was reminded that influenza CVVs are crucial for the production of influenza vaccines and that CVVs derived from zoonotic or novel human viruses require safety testing. Animal tests are variable and the currently used outbred ferret model is no exception when used for the comparison of CVVs and wild-type parental virus. Despite the requirement for CVVs to be attenuated compared to wild-type viruses, there are at present no independent criteria or parameters for the designation of "attenuated" other than direct comparison with wild-type virus. In addition, any delay in acquiring the wild-type virus for testing could hold up the release of a much needed CVV.

The proposed virus pathogenicity standards are intended to benchmark the ferret pathogenicity test, help in developing cut-offs and/or ranges for pathogenicity (and thus for attenuation) and to avoid the need for wild-type viruses for each and every CVV. It is expected that the use of such pathogenicity standards will simplify the production of CVVs without compromising safety. Standard viruses will be used occasionally to demonstrate the robustness of the test and to validate the established cut-offs and ranges. The development of robust pathology parameters will also aid in the training of newly qualified research staff.

The collection of ferret safety testing data from three CVV-producing laboratories is continuing and attempts are being made to define common parameters of attenuation. Potential parameters for evaluating attenuation include virus titres in the lung, mean weight loss, signs of disease, and virus in organs other than the respiratory tract. Based on 29 tested CVVs, results below the cut-off values for virus titres in the lungs of infected ferrets and for mean body weight loss appear to be markers of attenuation. It is currently unclear if lung pathology was similarly predictive and the scoring of this would need to be standardized. Virus titres in nasal washings and turbinates were found not to be predictive of attenuation.

In conclusion, despite the inherent variability of ferret tests, data obtained so far indicate that defining attenuation thresholds for some parameters may be possible. It may be that the use of a combination of parameters would have greater predictive power. The development of the proposed pathogenicity standards therefore remains feasible, and a collaborative study of one model attenuated virus and one model pathogenic virus is planned for 2019.

The Committee noted the project outcomes to date. During discussion, questions were asked about the cleanliness of test ferrets with respect to infectious agents and whether this might impact test outcomes. More work is clearly required on the development and use of standard viruses in the assessment of CVV attenuation but the Committee considered this to be a promising area of enquiry and looked forward to receiving further updates in due course.

9.2.2 Update on the development of the proposed First WHO International Standard for antibody to the influenza virus haemagglutinin stem domain

Following its endorsement in 2017 of the proposal to develop a First WHO International Standard for antibody to the influenza virus haemagglutinin stem domain, the Committee was provided with an update on the progress made during the initial exploratory phase of the project. The Committee was reminded that considerable efforts were being made to develop the next generation of influenza vaccines, some of which are intended to induce antibodies directed at the stem region of the HA molecule. Such vaccines were expected to be more broadly protective. HA stem-specific antibodies are measured using a range of functional and binding assays, and the standardization of serological results from clinical vaccine trials would allow for the comparison of trial outcomes, and potentially to the definition of generic correlates of protection. The proposed WHO international standard would be used to: (a) standardize the measurement of antibodies binding to the HA stem domain; (b) aid vaccine development by making results more comparable; and (c) aid in the defining of immunological correlates of protection for the next generation influenza vaccines.

The proposal comprised two phases – first, an initial small study would be conducted to evaluate potential materials and then a larger collaborative study would be carried out using freeze-dried candidate materials, ideally including samples from human clinical trials. The Committee was informed that funding for the preliminary work had been obtained from the Bill & Melinda Gates Foundation and a postdoctoral scientist recruited for the project. It was intended that the candidate material should consist of a pool of human sera containing antibodies reactive to the HA stem domain of Group 1 HA. The testing of individual human serum samples had now started with one high IgG titre pool (with considerable levels of IgA antibodies) having already been obtained. Next steps would include the selection of relevant assays for measuring antibodies to the HA stem domain and assessment of the ability of the pooled serum sample to reduce inter-laboratory variability. If successful, this will result in an application for funding to produce candidate standard(s), establish their characteristics and conduct the larger-scale collaborative study. It was expected that a workshop would be held to discuss the best way forward.

The Committee noted the progress made in this interesting project, endorsed its continuation and looked forward to receiving further updates in due course.

9.2.3 Proposed universal reagents for potency testing of inactivated poliomyelitis vaccines

The potency of IPV is based on the measurement of D-Ag and is a mandatory test in the WHO Recommendations to assure the quality, safety and efficacy of poliomyelitis vaccines (inactivated). D-Ag ELISA is currently the only approved test for measuring the D-Ag antigen content of IPV. The Committee was informed that despite more than 60 years of IPV manufacture, potency testing remained suboptimal, with all of the laboratories that had participated in the WHO collaborative study to develop the current WHO international standard using a different assay. In addition, both monoclonal and polyclonal antibodies had been used in different combinations – in some cases in assays subsequently discovered to be unsuitable for testing sIPV.

The current shortage of IPV has prompted the development of numerous new sIPV products, especially in LMIC following facilitation by WHO and other international agencies. With the proliferation of IPV manufacturers, some planning to produce sIPV, there is now an urgent need for harmonization. In this respect, the development of well-validated common ELISA reagents suitable for the testing of both conventional IPV and sIPV would be very helpful as this would allow for further harmonization of testing. In addition, there would be no need for every manufacturer and NCL to undertake the tedious process of validation and revalidation of their own reagents. This would be especially important to new sIPV manufacturers and would likely expedite the development and licensure of such vaccines. The results obtained in different laboratories would also be expected to be more consistent and comparable.

The Committee was informed that a joint project sponsored by PATH and the Bill & Melinda Gates Foundation will seek to address this need by providing a universal platform for the potency testing of all IPVs. The project will evaluate both human mAbs and mouse mAbs for use in IPV potency testing, optimize the technical protocol and validate the materials against both conventional IPV and sIPV. The project will involve an international collaborative study open to all vaccine manufacturers and NCLs. Although still at an early stage, a significant amount of preparatory work had been done, including evaluation of the analytical parameters of human and mouse mAbs and demonstration of the suitability of the proposed ELISA for the quantification of D antigen in conventional IPV and sIPV. Next steps will include the generation of stably transformed Chinese hamster ovary cell lines to produce sufficiently large quantities of the human and mouse mAbs for distribution to all interested laboratories.

The Committee endorsed the proposal (WHO/BS /2018.2342) to develop universal reagents for IPV testing. However, the issue of potential patent and ethical considerations regarding the source of human-donated biological materials was raised. It was felt that this was unlikely to present a problem in this case as there was an expectation that both PATH and the Bill & Melinda Gates Foundation would, as sponsors of the project, have already looked into the matter.

9.2.4 Proposed First WHO International Standard for anti EV-D68 serum

EV-D68 is an EV spread via the respiratory route that primarily causes respiratory disease. However, it is also associated with the neurological condition acute flaccid myelitis. The frequency of detection of EV-D68 infections has increased globally since the early 2000s and it is now recognized as a re-emerging pathogen. In 2014, 691 cases were reported in the USA spread across 46 states. These had resulted in severe respiratory illness in children and several fatalities. With the increasing global prevalence of the virus, the development of vaccines against

EV-D68 was becoming a priority, and there was thus a need for a WHO international standard for anti EV-D68 serum.

The proposed international standard would be used for the standardization of assays used in the evaluation and control testing of anti-EV-D68 vaccines and for general research. Envisaged users included industry, quality control laboratories and research laboratories investigating EV-D68. It was expected that source materials would be obtained from China and Europe towards the end of 2018, with filling and characterization taking place during the first half of 2019. A collaborative study would then be conducted in late 2019 with submission of its outcomes to the Committee in 2020.

The Committee endorsed the proposal (WHO/BS/2018.2342) to develop a First WHO International Standard for anti EV-D68 serum.

Annex 1

WHO Recommendations, Guidelines and other documents related to the manufacture, quality control and evaluation of biological substances used in medicine

WHO Recommendations, Guidelines and other documents are intended to provide guidance to those responsible for the production of biological substances as well as to others who may have to decide upon appropriate methods of assay and control to ensure that products are safe, reliable and potent. WHO Recommendations (previously called Requirements) and Guidelines are scientific and advisory in nature but may be adopted by an NRA as national requirements or used as the basis of such requirements.

Recommendations concerned with biological substances used in medicine are formulated by international groups of experts and are published in the WHO Technical Report Series[10] as listed below. A historical list of Requirements and other sets of Recommendations is available on request from the World Health Organization, 20 avenue Appia, 1211 Geneva 27, Switzerland. Reports of the WHO Expert Committee on Biological Standardization published in the WHO Technical Report Series can be purchased from:

WHO Press
World Health Organization
20 avenue Appia
1211 Geneva 27
Switzerland
Telephone: + 41 22 791 3246
Fax: +41 22 791 4857
Email: bookorders@who.int
Website: www.who.int/bookorders

Individual Recommendations and Guidelines may be obtained free of charge as offprints by writing to:

Technologies Standards and Norms
Department of Essential Medicines and Health Products
World Health Organization
20 avenue Appia
1211 Geneva 27
Switzerland

---

[10] Abbreviated in the following pages to "TRS".

Recommendations, Guidelines and other documents	Reference
Animal cells, use of, as in vitro substrates for the production of biologicals	Revised 2010, TRS 978 (2013)
BCG vaccines (dried)	Revised 2011, TRS 979 (2013)
Biological products: good manufacturing practices	Revised 2015, TRS 999 (2016)
Biological standardization and control: a scientific review commissioned by the UK National Biological Standards Board (1997)	Unpublished document WHO/BLG/97.1
Biological substances: International Standards and Reference Reagents	Revised 2004, TRS 932 (2006)
Biotherapeutic products, changes to approved biotherapeutic products: procedures and data requirements	Adopted 2017, TRS 1011 (2018)
Biotherapeutic products, similar	Adopted 2009, TRS 977 (2013)
Biotherapeutic products, similar: WHO Questions and Answers[11]	Adopted 2018; online document
Biotherapeutic protein products prepared by recombinant DNA technology	Revised 2013, TRS 987 (2014); Addendum 2015, TRS 999 (2016)
Blood, blood components and plasma derivatives: collection, processing and quality control	Revised 1992, TRS 840 (1994)
Blood and blood components: management as essential medicines	Adopted 2016, TRS 1004 (2017)
Blood components and plasma: estimation of residual risk of HIV, HBV or HCV infections	Adopted 2016, TRS 1004 (2017)
Blood establishments: good manufacturing practices	Adopted 2010, TRS 961 (2011)
Blood plasma (human) for fractionation	Adopted 2005, TRS 941 (2007)
Blood plasma products (human): viral inactivation and removal procedures	Adopted 2001, TRS 924 (2004)
Blood regulatory systems, assessment criteria for national	Adopted 2011, TRS 979 (2013)

---

[11] Available online at: https://www.who.int/biologicals/biotherapeutics/similar_biotherapeutic_products/en/

Recommendations, Guidelines and other documents	Reference
Cholera vaccines (inactivated, oral)	Adopted 2001, TRS 924 (2004)
Dengue tetravalent vaccines (live, attenuated)	Revised 2011, TRS 979 (2013)
Diphtheria, tetanus, pertussis (whole cell), and combined (DTwP) vaccines	Revised 2012, TRS 980 (2014)
Diphtheria vaccines (adsorbed)	Revised 2012, TRS 980 (2014)
DNA vaccines: assuring quality and nonclinical safety	Revised 2005, TRS 941 (2007)
Ebola vaccines	Adopted 2017, TRS 1011 (2018)
Haemophilus influenzae type b conjugate vaccines	Revised 1998, TRS 897 (2000)
Haemorrhagic fever with renal syndrome (HFRS) vaccines (inactivated)	Adopted 1993, TRS 848 (1994)
Hepatitis A vaccines (inactivated)	Adopted 1994, TRS 858 (1995)
Hepatitis B vaccines prepared from plasma	Revised 1987, TRS 771 (1988)
Hepatitis B vaccines (recombinant)	Revised 2010, TRS 978 (2013)
Hepatitis E vaccines (recombinant)	Adopted 2018, TRS 1016 (2019)
Human immunodeficiency virus rapid diagnostic tests for professional use and/or self-testing Technical Specifications Series for WHO Prequalification – Diagnostic Assessment	Adopted 2017, TRS 1011 (2018)
Human interferons prepared from lymphoblastoid cells	Adopted 1988, TRS 786 (1989)
Influenza vaccines (inactivated)	Revised 2003, TRS 927 (2005)
Influenza vaccines (inactivated): labelling information for use in pregnant women	Addendum to TRS 927; TRS 1004 (2017)
Influenza vaccines (live)	Revised 2009, TRS 977 (2013)
Influenza vaccines, human, pandemic: regulatory preparedness	Adopted 2007, TRS 963 (2011)
Influenza vaccines, human, pandemic: regulatory preparedness in non-vaccine-producing countries	Adopted 2016, TRS 1004 (2017)
Influenza vaccines, human, pandemic: safe development and production	Adopted 2018, TRS 1016 (2019)

Recommendations, Guidelines and other documents	Reference
In vitro diagnostic medical devices, establishing stability of, Technical Guidance Series for WHO Prequalification – Diagnostic Assessment	Adopted 2017, TRS 1011 (2018)
Japanese encephalitis vaccines (inactivated) for human use	Revised 2007, TRS 963 (2011)
Japanese encephalitis vaccines (live, attenuated) for human use	Revised 2012, TRS 980 (2014)
Louse-borne human typhus vaccines (live)	Adopted 1982, TRS 687 (1983)
Malaria vaccines (recombinant)	Adopted 2012, TRS 980 (2014)
Measles, mumps and rubella vaccines and combined vaccines (live)	Adopted 1992, TRS 848 (1994);
Meningococcal polysaccharide vaccines	Adopted 1975, TRS 594 (1976); Addendum 1980, TRS 658 (1981); Amendment 1999, TRS 904 (2002)
Meningococcal A conjugate vaccines	Adopted 2006, TRS 962 (2011)
Meningococcal C conjugate vaccines	Adopted 2001, TRS 924 (2004); Addendum (revised) 2007, TRS 963 (2011)
Monoclonal antibodies	Adopted 1991, TRS 822 (1992)
Monoclonal antibodies as similar biotherapeutic products	Adopted 2016, TRS 1004 (2017)
Papillomavirus vaccines (human, recombinant, virus-like particle)	Revised 2015, TRS 999 (2016)
Pertussis vaccines (acellular)	Revised 2011, TRS 979 (2013)
Pertussis vaccines (whole-cell)	Revised 2005, TRS 941 (2007)
Pharmaceutical products, storage and transport of time- and temperature-sensitive	Adopted 2010, TRS 961 (2011)
Pneumococcal conjugate vaccines	Revised 2009, TRS 977 (2013)
Poliomyelitis vaccines (inactivated)	Revised 2014, TRS 993 (2015)
Poliomyelitis vaccines: safe production and quality control	Revised 2018, TRS 1016 (2019)
Poliomyelitis vaccines (oral)	Revised 2012, TRS 980 (2014)

Recommendations, Guidelines and other documents	Reference
Quality assurance for biological products, guidelines for national authorities	Adopted 1991, TRS 822 (1992)
Rabies vaccines for human use (inactivated) produced in cell substrates and embryonated eggs	Revised 2005, TRS 941 (2007)
Reference materials, secondary: for NAT-based and antigen assays: calibration against WHO International Standards	Adopted 2016, TRS 1004 (2017)
Regulation and licensing of biological products in countries with newly developing regulatory authorities	Adopted 1994, TRS 858 (1995)
Regulatory risk evaluation on finding an adventitious agent in a marketed vaccine: scientific principles	Adopted 2014, TRS 993 (2015)
Rotavirus vaccines (live, attenuated, oral)	Adopted 2005, TRS 941 (2007)
Smallpox vaccines	Revised 2003, TRS 926 (2004)
Snake antivenom immunoglobulins	Revised 2016, TRS 1004 (2017)
Sterility of biological substances	Revised 1973, TRS 530 (1973); Amendment 1995, TRS 872 (1998)
Synthetic peptide vaccines	Adopted 1997, TRS 889 (1999)
Tetanus vaccines (adsorbed)	Revised 2012, TRS 980 (2014)
Thiomersal for vaccines: regulatory expectations for elimination, reduction or removal	Adopted 2003, TRS 926 (2004)
Thromboplastins and plasma used to control oral anticoagulant therapy	Revised 2011, TRS 979 (2013)
Tick-borne encephalitis vaccines (inactivated)	Adopted 1997, TRS 889 (1999)
Transmissible spongiform encephalopathies in relation to biological and pharmaceutical products[12]	Revised 2005, WHO (2006)
Tuberculins	Revised 1985, TRS 745 (1987)
Typhoid vaccines, conjugated	Adopted 2013, TRS 987 (2014)

---

[12] Available online at: http://www.who.int/biologicals/publications/en/whotse2003.pdf

Recommendations, Guidelines and other documents	Reference
Typhoid vaccines (live, attenuated, Ty21a, oral)	Adopted 1983, TRS 700 (1984)
Typhoid vaccines, Vi polysaccharide	Adopted 1992, TRS 840 (1994)
Vaccines, changes to approved vaccines: procedures and data requirements	Adopted 2014, TRS 993 (2015)
Vaccines, clinical evaluation: regulatory expectations	Revised 2016, TRS 1004 (2017)
Vaccines, clinical evaluation: use of human challenge trials	Adopted 2016, TRS 1004 (2017)
Vaccines, lot release	Adopted 2010, TRS 978 (2013)
Vaccines, nonclinical evaluation	Adopted 2003, TRS 926 (2004)
Vaccines, nonclinical evaluation of vaccine adjuvants and adjuvanted vaccines	Adopted 2013, TRS 987 (2014)
Vaccines, prequalification procedure	Adopted 2010, TRS 978 (2013)
Vaccines, stability evaluation	Adopted 2006, TRS 962 (2011)
Vaccines, stability evaluation for use under extended controlled temperature conditions	Adopted 2015, TRS 999 (2016)
Varicella vaccines (live)	Revised 1993, TRS 848 (1994)
Yellow fever vaccines	Revised 2010, TRS 978 (2013)
Yellow fever vaccines, laboratories approved by WHO for the production of	Revised 1995, TRS 872 (1998)
Yellow fever virus, production and testing of WHO primary seed lot 213-77 and reference batch 168-736	Adopted 1985, TRS 745 (1987)

Annex 2

Recommendations to assure the quality, safety and efficacy of recombinant hepatitis E vaccines

Recommendations published by the World Health Organization (WHO) are intended to be scientific and advisory in nature. Each of the following sections constitutes recommendations for national regulatory authorities (NRAs) and for manufacturers of biological products. If an NRA so desires, these WHO Recommendations may be adopted as definitive national requirements, or modifications may be justified and made by the NRA. It is recommended that modifications to these WHO Recommendations are made only on condition that such modifications ensure that the product is at least as safe and efficacious as that prepared in accordance with the recommendations set out below. The parts of each section printed in small type are comments or examples intended to provide additional guidance to manufacturers and NRAs.

Abbreviations

ALT	alanine aminotransferase
DNA	deoxyribonucleic acid
ECBS	WHO Expert Committee on Biological Standardization
ELISA	enzyme-linked immunosorbent assay
GACVS	WHO Global Advisory Committee on Vaccine Safety
GLP	good laboratory practice(s)
HEV	hepatitis E virus
HIV	human immunodeficiency virus
HPLC	high-performance liquid chromatography
HPSEC	high-performance size-exclusion chromatography
IFA	immunofluorescence foci assay
IgG	immunoglobulin G
IgM	immunoglobulin M
LMIC	low- and middle-income countries
MALDI-TOF	matrix-assisted laser desorption/ionization time-of-flight mass spectrometry
MCB	master cell bank
NAT	nucleic acid amplification technique
NCL	national control laboratory
NRA	national regulatory authority
ORF2	open reading frame 2
PCR	polymerase chain reaction
RNA	ribonucleic acid
SAGE	WHO Strategic Advisory Group of Experts on Immunization
SDS-PAGE	sodium dodecyl sulfate polyacrylamide gel electrophoresis
TEM	transmission electron microscopy
ULN	upper limit of normal
WCB	working cell bank

Introduction

Hepatitis E virus (HEV) is a major cause of sporadic and epidemic hepatitis, and is found worldwide. The highest seroprevalence rates are observed in regions where low standards of sanitation increase the risk of virus transmission (*1*).

The WHO Strategic Advisory Group of Experts on Immunization (SAGE) issued a position paper in 2015 which reviewed existing evidence on the burden of hepatitis E and on the safety, immunogenicity, efficacy and cost-effectiveness of a hepatitis E vaccine that was first licensed in China (*1*). This vaccine contains the HEV open reading frame 2 (ORF2) capsid protein, corresponding to amino acids 368–606 of ORF2, manufactured in *Escherichia coli* using recombinant technology. The WHO Global Advisory Committee on Vaccine Safety (GACVS) had reviewed this same hepatitis E vaccine in 2014 and concluded that it had an acceptable safety profile (*2*). In 2016, WHO published its *Global health sector strategy on viral hepatitis 2016–2021* (*3*), which addresses hepatitis A, B, C and E. Hepatitis E is probably the most neglected of the four. This strategy document highlights the urgent need to address all viral hepatitis, including hepatitis E for which only one vaccine is approved anywhere in the world and for which no effective therapies exist.

Following requests from manufacturers and other stakeholders for WHO to develop Recommendations to assure the quality, safety and efficacy of recombinant hepatitis E vaccines, a series of meetings was convened by WHO to review the current status of development and likely time to licensure of such vaccines (*4*). These meetings were attended by experts from around the world involved in the research, manufacture, regulatory assessment and approval, control-testing and release of hepatitis E vaccines. Participants were drawn from academia, national regulatory authorities (NRAs), national control laboratories (NCLs) and industry.

Purpose and scope

These WHO Recommendations provide guidance to NRAs and manufacturers on the manufacturing processes, and nonclinical and clinical evaluations, needed to assure the quality, safety and efficacy of recombinant hepatitis E vaccines.

The document encompasses recombinant hepatitis E vaccines for prophylactic use based on the ORF2 capsid protein.

The document should be read in conjunction with other relevant WHO guidance, especially on the nonclinical (*5*) and clinical (*6*) evaluation of vaccines. Other WHO guidance should also be considered, including – as appropriate to the vaccine – guidance on the evaluation of animal cell cultures as substrates for the manufacture of biological medicinal products and for the characterization

WHO Technical Report Series, No. 1016, 2019

of cell banks (*7*) and on the nonclinical evaluation of vaccine adjuvants and adjuvanted vaccines (*8*).

Terminology

The definitions given below apply to the terms as used in these WHO Recommendations. These terms may have different meanings in other contexts.

Adventitious agents: contaminating microorganisms that may include bacteria, fungi, mycoplasmas, and endogenous and exogenous viruses that have been unintentionally introduced into the manufacturing process.

Cell bank: a collection of containers containing aliquots of a suspension of cells from a single pool of uniform composition, stored frozen under defined conditions (typically −60 °C or below for yeast or bacteria and in liquid nitrogen for insect or mammalian cell lines). The terms **master cell bank** (MCB) and **working cell bank** (WCB) are used in these Recommendations. An MCB is a bank of a cell substrate representing a well-characterized collection of cells derived from a single tissue or cell, and from which all subsequent cell banks used for vaccine production will be derived. A WCB is a cell bank derived by propagation of cells from an MCB under defined conditions, and is used to initiate production of cell cultures on a lot-by-lot basis. The WCB is also referred to as a "manufacturer's working cell bank" in other documents.

> The individual containers (for example, ampoules or vials) should be representative of the pool of cells from which they are taken and should be frozen on the same day following the same procedure and using the same equipment and reagents.

Cell substrate: cells used to manufacture a biological product.

Final bulk: the formulated vaccine present in a container from which the final containers are filled. The final bulk may be prepared from one or more **purified antigen bulks**. Mixing should result in a uniform preparation to ensure that the final containers are homogenous.

Final filled lot: a collection of sealed final containers of finished vaccine that is homogeneous with respect to the risk of contamination during the filling process. All of the final containers must therefore have been filled from a single vessel of final bulk in one working session. Also referred to as "final lot" or "final product" in other documents.

Purified antigen bulk: the processed, purified antigen that has been prepared from either a single harvest or from a pool of single harvests. It is the parent material from which the final bulk is prepared.

Recombinant DNA technology: technology that joins together (that is, recombines) DNA segments from two or more different DNA molecules that are inserted into a host organism to produce new genetic combinations. It is also referred to as "gene modification" or "genetic engineering" because the original gene is synthetically altered and changed. These new genes, when inserted into the expression system, form the basis for the production of recombinant DNA-derived protein(s).

Seed lot (master, working seed lot): a quantity of bacterial, viral or cell suspension that has been derived from one strain, has been processed as a single lot and has a uniform composition. It is used to prepare the inoculum for the production medium.

Single harvest: the biological material prepared from a single production run before further downstream processing.

Single harvest pool: a pool of a number of single harvests of the same virus type processed at the same time.

General considerations

Hepatitis E virus

HEV is a non-enveloped positive-sense RNA virus of the Hepeviridae family. The single-stranded viral genome is 7.2 kb in length and contains three open reading frames. Of these, ORF2 codes for the viral capsid protein which is the target of neutralizing antibodies against HEV (9). HEV isolates were classified into four human genotypes (genotypes 1–4) such that the nucleic acid variation of ORF2 between different genotypes is more than 20%; however, the four genotypes form a single serotype based on their immune reactivity. Different genotypes differ by more than 8.8% in highly conserved ORF1 and ORF2 amino acid sequences (10). The genotypes have been subdivided further into numerous subtypes – though the underlying criteria are controversial (11, 12). Nevertheless, HEV strains that infect humans belong to one currently identifiable serotype, with marked serological cross-reactivity as well as evidence for cross-protection in non-human primates and in humans (13). New genotypes of HEV (that is, genotypes 5–8), with limited information on their pathogenicity in humans and their cross-reactivity with human genotypes 1–4, were reported during the development of these WHO Recommendations (14).

Epidemiology

Almost all of the information available on the epidemiology of HEV concerns genotypes 1–4. HEV genotypes 1 and 2 primarily infect humans, whereas genotypes 3 and 4 mainly infect mammalian animals with occasional cross-species transmission to humans.

The epidemiology and clinical presentation of HEV infection vary greatly by geographical location, due primarily to differences in circulating HEV genotypes (15–17). A global burden of disease study estimated that in 2005 HEV

WHO Technical Report Series, No. 1016, 2019

genotypes 1 and 2 accounted for approximately 20.1 million HEV infections, 3.4 million symptomatic cases, 70 000 deaths, and 3000 stillbirths (*18*).

Hepatitis E infection due to genotypes 1 and 2 has been identified in at least 63 countries, of which around half have reported large outbreaks (*18*). The overall burden of disease due to hepatitis E is greatest in low- and middle-income countries (LMIC), especially where clean drinking-water is scarce, as faecal contamination of drinking-water is a major route of HEV transmission (*18*). Although there is no evidence of large outbreaks of hepatitis E occurring in developed countries, small clusters of cases associated with foodborne transmission have occurred in Europe and Japan (*19*). There are also countries with no recorded sporadic disease or outbreaks but where serological evidence of past HEV infection has been reported, suggesting that HEV infection may be endemic.

Waterborne hepatitis E outbreaks have been reported from at least 30 countries on three continents – Africa, Asia and North America (Mexico) – and have been caused chiefly by HEV genotype 1. Large waterborne hepatitis E outbreaks frequently occur in the Indian subcontinent (*20*). In Australia, Europe and North America, cases due to genotype 1 have been reported in returning travellers. Determining the distribution of HEV genotype 2 has proved difficult, with most cases reported from Mexico, Namibia, Nigeria and several other West African countries. However, such infections seem rare with only a few cases reported to date (*21–23*).

In recent years, there have been numerous outbreaks caused by HEV genotype 1 in camps for internally displaced persons and refugees in Africa. There is some evidence that other modes of transmission (including from person to person) may contribute to the prolongation of outbreaks, particularly in displaced populations (*24*). Recent large outbreaks have occurred among displaced persons in Chad, Niger, Sudan and Uganda (*21, 25–27*). The first serologically confirmed outbreak documented in Africa occurred among Angolan refugees in Namibia in 1983. During a recent outbreak in northern Uganda, a high mortality rate was recorded among children under 2 years of age (*25*); however, the cause of death in these children was not verified. As was the case in northern Uganda, an outbreak in South Sudan also started during the rainy season, with high disease attack rates (7.4%) observed among camp residents, and high levels of mortality recorded among pregnant women (10.4%) (*26*). A sero-survey conducted during this outbreak showed that more than half of the camp residents had no evidence of current or past HEV infection, suggesting that these individuals remained uninfected. Both the Ugandan and South Sudanese outbreaks lasted well over a year, indicating that the implementing of prevention and control efforts during such outbreaks can be challenging.

Although waterborne hepatitis E outbreaks can result in large numbers of cases over a short period of time, most hepatitis E cases in LMIC probably occur within smaller clusters or result from sporadic transmission (*28*). The risk factors for sporadic hepatitis E are less well understood, although water contamination may play a role.

In developed countries, where the hepatitis E disease burden is much lower, zoonotic transmission, primarily through the consumption of uncooked or undercooked meat, is a potential mode of transmission; with HEV genotype 3 being the predominant genotype (*16*). Despite the ubiquity of HEV genotype 3 in the domestic pig population, clinically apparent human infections with this genotype have been reported almost entirely in developed countries.

In recent years, HEV genotype 4 has been found to circulate in animals in China, India and several European countries; with most human cases of hepatitis due to HEV genotype 4 having been reported in China. The main mode of transmission of HEV genotype 4 is also believed to be the consumption of infected pork and contact with domestic pigs.

There is no evidence of the sexual transmission of HEV (*16*). Although transfusion-associated HEV transmission occurs and is well documented, its contribution to the overall disease burden is limited (*16, 29, 30*).

Disease and diagnosis

HEV-infected individuals exhibit a wide clinical spectrum, ranging from asymptomatic infection through acute icteric hepatitis to fulminant hepatitis. Asymptomatic infection is common in immunocompetent individuals and the disease presentation is often mild. The ratio of symptomatic to asymptomatic infection has been estimated to range from 1:2 to 1:10 or more in outbreak settings and may be dependent on age at infection. HEV infection occurs in children and the probability of symptomatic disease increases with age (*1, 31*). The incubation period ranges from 15 to 60 days, with a mean of 40 days (*32*). Although infection with HEV genotype 1 is associated with serious disease more often than infection with other genotypes, the extent to which such severe disease occurs with genotypes 2 and 4 is not well documented. Studies in non-human primates have shown a relationship between the dose of viral inoculum and the host's immunological response and degree of liver injury (*33*).

In LMIC, where HEV genotypes 1 and, to a lesser extent, 2 are the most commonly identified causes of hepatitis E, the disease mainly affects young adults (for example, those aged 15–39 years), with a preponderance in males. During waterborne outbreaks, children may develop severe hepatitis E due to coinfection with hepatitis A virus (*34*).

Fulminating hepatitis E occurs at a disproportionately high rate among pregnant women during epidemics (*35–37*), the disease being typically most severe during the third trimester of pregnancy (*38, 39*). While mortality from hepatitis E ranges from 0.1% to 4% in the general population, it can range from 10% to 50% among women in the third trimester of pregnancy (*1, 38, 40, 41*). The mechanism underlying the high mortality rate among pregnant women is unclear (*31*). Causes of death include fulminant liver failure and obstetric complications, including excessive bleeding (*36*). HEV can be transmitted from mother to fetus during pregnancy, resulting in poor fetal outcomes that include miscarriage, premature delivery and stillbirths (*20, 35*).

HEV genotypes 3 and 4 have been repeatedly reported to cause severe disease as well as chronic hepatitis E in immunocompromised people in China and Europe. Chronic infections do not occur in otherwise healthy individuals. HEV infection in those who receive immunosuppressive treatment following solid organ or bone marrow transplantation, and in those with severe immunodeficiency of other origins, is associated with risk of progression to chronic hepatitis E (*42*). HIV-infected patients are not at higher risk for HEV infection; the number of acute infections reported in these populations is low and very few chronic cases have been reported (*43–45*). The clinical manifestation and progression of chronic hepatitis E (lasting > 6 months) are variable with some cases progressing to significant fibrosis in a relatively short period of time.

Recently, a single case of chronic infection with camelid HEV (which is HEV genotype 7) was reported in a patient who had undergone liver transplantation and who regularly consumed camel meat and milk – suggesting that this genotype might infect humans via foodborne zoonotic transmission. It was reported that immunoglobulin G (IgG) and immunoglobulin M (IgM) antibodies against new HEV genotypes can be detected by HEV genotype 1 antigen (*46*).

Individuals with pre-existing chronic liver disease are prone to developing severe hepatitis following HEV infection. Those with advanced liver disease, including cirrhosis, may develop acute hepatic failure when infected with HEV (*20*). The burden of HEV-induced acute liver failure in patients with pre-existing chronic liver disease is unknown.

Laboratory diagnosis of recent HEV infection is based on the detection of HEV-specific IgM antibodies, the recent appearance or several-fold increase in titres of specific IgG antibodies or the detection of HEV RNA in blood samples (*47*). Specific detection of HEV antigen can also be a marker for the diagnosis of hepatitis E (*48*). However, the performance characteristics (sensitivity and specificity) of some currently available commercial assays for anti-HEV antibodies are suboptimal (*49–55*). In one study that compared six different assays the sensitivity of the individual assays ranged from 72% to 98%, and specificity from 78% to 96%; furthermore, the kappa coefficients for agreement between the results of various pairs of tests varied from 0.42 to 0.80 (*56*). This has implications for clinical trials based on serological outcomes and for studies that rely on these serological tests to estimate the burden of disease and previous history of infection. One recent study compared the results obtained using a newer diagnostic assay to the results obtained from the assay used in the original study of seroprevalence in rural Bangladesh and found that the newer assay showed much higher seroprevalence in the population (*57*).

Immune response to natural HEV infection

Past HEV infection is characterized by the presence of serum IgG antibodies directed against the viral capsid protein, which may confer protection against reinfection. However, the protective IgG antibody concentration is not known and the duration of protection following natural infection is uncertain. In Kashmir, serological follow-up of 45 individuals known to have had hepatitis E during the 1978 outbreak found that 47% had detectable anti-HEV IgG 14 years after infection (*58*) – though the difficulties in interpreting serological assay results mentioned above should be noted. A recent study based on 67 months of serological follow-up data and mathematical modelling suggested that naturally acquired anti-HEV IgG will remain detectable in half of seropositive individuals for 14.5 years (*59*). In another follow-up study, 100% of people had measurable anti-HEV IgG 5 years after infection (*60*). However, the subjects studied were living in hyperendemic areas where the possibility of multiple re-exposures and natural boosting cannot be ruled out.

There is some evidence that naturally acquired HEV infection does not confer lifelong immunity. For example, even in endemic areas, the prevalence of anti-HEV IgG in the population does not reach the very high levels observed for hepatitis A which does confer lifelong protection, and attack rates are highest among young to middle-aged adults, suggesting that infection during early life may not confer lifelong protection, or that infections usually occur later in life. In addition, outbreaks recur in countries where previous epidemics would be expected to have resulted in a level of population immunity sufficient to prevent future outbreaks. The duration of protection conferred by naturally acquired antibodies has important implications for long-term vaccine efficacy.

Vaccines against HEV

Although many experimental hepatitis E vaccines have been evaluated in virus challenge studies in non-human primates, other animal models or clinical trials, only one vaccine has been licensed for human use as of mid-2018. This vaccine was licensed in China in December 2011 for use in people aged 16 years and over. It is based on a 239-amino-acid recombinant HEV peptide, corresponding to amino acids 368–606 of ORF2 which encodes the capsid protein of genotype 1

HEV (*61–64*). Vaccine efficacy after three doses was 100% over a 12-month period after the last dose, and 95.5% over 19 months in all subjects who had received at least one dose. Other vaccines based on the HEV capsid protein are currently in nonclinical or clinical development.

International reference materials

Subsequent sections of this document refer to WHO reference materials that may be used in laboratory or clinical evaluations. Key standards used in the control of hepatitis E vaccines include the following:

- A WHO reference preparation for antibodies to hepatitis E virus is available for the standardization of diagnostic tests for use in seroprevalence studies and for assessing immunity. This WHO interim Reference Reagent for hepatitis E virus antibody, human serum (code 95/584) was established by the WHO Expert Committee on Biological Standardization (ECBS) in 1997 and was assigned a unitage of 50 units/ampoule (*65*). The preparation is held and distributed by the National Institute for Biological Standards and Control (NIBSC), Potters Bar, the United Kingdom.

- WHO international reference preparations for hepatitis E virus RNA are also available. These standards are suitable for the calibration of in-house or working standards for use in the amplification and detection of hepatitis E virus RNA. The First WHO International Standard for hepatitis E virus RNA for NAT-based assays was established by the ECBS in 2011 and was assigned a unitage of 250 000 IU/ml (*66*). The First WHO International Reference Panel for hepatitis E virus genotypes for NAT-based assays (code 8578/13) contains 11 members and was established by the ECBS in 2015 (*67*). These two preparations are held and distributed by the Paul-Ehrlich-Institut (PEI), Langen, Germany.

- A product-specific national reference for use in potency assays is under development by the National Institutes for Food and Drug Control (NIFDC), China.

The WHO Catalogue of International Reference Preparations should be consulted for the latest list of appropriate WHO international standards and other reference materials. See: http://www.who.int/bloodproducts/catalogue/en/.

Part A. Manufacturing recommendations

A.1 Definitions

A.1.1 International name and proper name

The international name should be "recombinant hepatitis E vaccine". The proper name should be the equivalent of the international name in the language of the country of origin.

The use of the international name should be limited to vaccines that meet the specifications elaborated below.

A.1.2 Descriptive definition

The recombinant hepatitis E vaccine is a sterile liquid vaccine preparation that contains purified recombinant capsid protein of hepatitis E virus. The protein may be formulated with a suitable adjuvant. Such vaccines are for prophylactic use.

A.2 General manufacturing recommendations

The general manufacturing recommendations contained in WHO good manufacturing practices for pharmaceutical products: main principles (68) and WHO good manufacturing practices for biological products (69) should apply to the design, establishment, operation, control and maintenance of manufacturing facilities for recombinant hepatitis E vaccines. The addition of any excipient should be justified, including preservative.

A.3 Control of source materials

A.3.1 Cells for antigen production

The use of any type of cell should be based on a cell bank system (7, 70) and should be approved by, and registered with, the NRA. The maximum allowable number of passages or population doublings from the MCB to production level should be approved by the NRA.

A.3.1.1 Recombinant cells for production

The history and characteristics of the parental cells, including bacteria or eukaryotic cells if relevant, should be fully described. The recombinant vaccine production strain (parental cell transformed with the recombinant expression construct) should be fully described and information should be given on the results of any adventitious agent testing required, and on the homogeneity and accuracy of the inserted sequence (including copy number per cell) for the MCB and WCB. Plasmid retention should be demonstrated as part of process validation. A full description of the biological characteristics of the host cell and expression strategy should be given. This should include genetic markers of the host cell, the construction, genetics and structure of the expression system, induction method, DNA sequencing of the insert and the origin and identification of the HEV sequence that is being cloned. The complete sequence of the entire construct should be determined, including control elements, and should be provided as part of the validation of the production process. The molecular and physiological measures used to promote and control the expression of the cloned HEV sequence in the host cell should be described in detail (*71*).

Cells must be maintained in a state that allows for recovery of viable cells without alteration of genotype (for example, frozen in liquid nitrogen). The cells should be recovered if necessary in selective media so that the genotype and phenotype are maintained and clearly identifiable. Cell banks should be identified and fully characterized using appropriate tests.

Data (for example, on plasmid restriction enzyme mapping, nutritional requirements or antibiotic resistance, if applicable) that demonstrate the genetic stability of the expression system during passage of the recombinant WCB up to and beyond the passage level used for production should be provided to, and approved by, the NRA as part of the validation of the production process. Any instability of the expression system occurring in the seed culture or after a production-scale run should be documented. Stability studies should also be performed to confirm cell viability, maintenance of the expression system etc. after retrieval from storage. These studies may be performed as part of their routine use in production or may involve samples being taken specifically for this purpose.

A.3.1.1.1 *Tests on recombinant bacteria MCB and WCB*

MCBs and WCBs (bacterial expression system) used for production should be tested to demonstrate that only the bacterial production strain is present in the MCB and WCB, and that contaminating bacteria and fungi are absent.

A.3.1.2 Other expression systems

If expression systems other than bacterial systems are used, characterization may be based on the WHO Recommendations to assure the quality, safety and efficacy of recombinant human papillomavirus virus-like particle vaccines (*72*), Recommendations for the evaluation of animal cell cultures as substrates for the manufacture of biological medicinal products and for the characterization of cell banks (*7*) and Guidelines on the quality, safety and efficacy of biotherapeutic protein products prepared by recombinant DNA technology (*71*).

MCBs and WCBs (animal cell culture system) used for production should be tested for the absence of bacterial, fungal and mycoplasmal contamination by appropriate tests, as specified in Part A, section 5.2 of the WHO General requirements for the sterility of biological substances (*73*) and its 1995 amendment for mycoplasma (*74*).

A.4

Control of HEV protein production

A.4.1

Microbial purity

The microbial purity of recombinant bacterial cultures should be monitored in each fermentation vessel at the end of the production run by methods approved by the NRA.

Any agent added to the fermenter or bioreactor with the intention of feeding cells or of inducing production or increasing cell density should be approved by the NRA. No antibiotics should be added at any stage of manufacturing unless approved by the NRA.

A.4.2

Control of single harvests

A.4.2.1

Storage and intermediate hold times

After the production run, the cell suspension or the product partially purified from it (for example, by preparation of inclusion bodies) should be maintained under conditions shown by the manufacturer to retain the desired biological activity. Hold times should be approved by the NRA.

A.4.2.2

Tests on single harvest or single harvest pool

If appropriate, tests may be conducted on a single antigen harvest or on a pool of single antigen harvests depending on the production strategy. The protocol should be approved by the NRA.

A.4.2.2.1 *Sampling*

Samples required for the testing of antigen harvests should be taken immediately on harvesting or pooling and before further processing. Tests for sterility and adventitious agents, as described below in sections A.4.2.2.2 and A.4.2.2.4 respectively, should preferably be performed within 24 hours. If these tests are not performed within 24 hours, the samples taken for these tests should be stored at an appropriate temperature. Where mammalian or insect cell expression systems are used, samples should be stored at $-60\,°C$ and subjected to no more than one freeze–thaw cycle. For other systems in which the infectivity of adventitious agents will not need to be preserved, an appropriate temperature should be chosen. Moreover, evidence should be provided that the freezing process does not affect the viability of the adventitious agents putatively present in the sample.

A.4.2.2.2 *Tests for bacteria, fungi and mycoplasmas*

Harvests from bacterial expression systems could have bacterial contamination. Therefore, a method such as the microbial limits test may be appropriate for addressing microbial purity. Such testing should be approved by the NRA.

For non-bacterial production systems, each single antigen harvest or single harvest pool should be shown to be free from bacterial, fungal and mycoplasmal contamination by appropriate tests, as specified in Part A, section 5.2 of the WHO General requirements for the sterility of biological substances (*73*) and its 1995 amendment for mycoplasma (*74*).

A.4.2.2.3 *Test for identity*

Each harvest should be identified as HEV antigen by a suitable assay such as sodium dodecyl sulfate polyacrylamide gel electrophoresis (SDS-PAGE), enzyme-linked immunosorbent assay (ELISA) or other methods. The tests should be approved by the NRA. Alternatively, the identity can be confirmed as part of testing of the purified antigen.

A.4.2.2.4 *Tests for adventitious agents if insect or mammalian cells are used in production*

Each single harvest or single harvest pool should be tested for adventitious viruses in cell cultures selected for their appropriateness to the origin and passage history of the insect cell substrate and recombinant baculovirus or the mammalian cell substrate. These cell cultures should include, as a minimum, a monkey kidney cell line and a human cell line. Antisera used for the purpose of neutralizing the recombinant baculovirus should be free from antibodies that may neutralize adventitious viruses and should preferably be generated by the immunization of specific-pathogen-free animals with an antigen made from a source (other than the production cell line) which has itself been tested for freedom from adventitious agents. The inoculated indicator cells should be examined microscopically for cytopathic changes. At the end of the examination period, the cells should also be tested for haemadsorbing viruses.

Additional testing for specific adventitious viruses may be performed (for example, using polymerase chain reaction (PCR) amplification techniques).

A.5　Control of purified antigen bulk

The purification process can be applied to a single antigen harvest, part of a single antigen harvest or a pool of single antigen harvests, and should be approved by the NRA. The maximum number of harvests that may be pooled should also be approved by the NRA. Adequate purification may require several purification steps based on different biophysical and/or biochemical principles and may involve disassembly and reassembly of particles. The entire process (sequence of process steps) used for the purification of the final antigen bulk should be appropriately validated and should be approved by the NRA. Any reagents added during the purification processes (such as DNase) should be documented and their removal adequately validated and tested for, as appropriate (see section A.5.1.7).

The purified antigen bulk can be stored under conditions shown by the manufacturer to allow it to retain the critical quality attributes. Intermediate hold times should be approved by the NRA.

A.5.1   Tests on the purified antigen bulk

Purified antigen bulks should be subjected to the tests listed below. Some tests may be omitted if performed on the adsorbed antigen bulk. All quality control release tests and specifications for purified antigen bulk, unless otherwise specified, should be validated by the manufacturer and approved by the NRA.

A.5.1.1   Purity

The degree of purity of the purified antigen bulk, and levels of residual host-cell protein and DNA, should be assessed by suitable methods. One suitable method for analysing the proportion of potential contaminating proteins is SDS-PAGE under reducing denaturing conditions. The protein bands within the gel should be identified by sensitive staining techniques and quantified by densitometric analysis. Other suitable methods such as high-performance liquid chromatography (HPLC) may also be used for purity analysis.

A.5.1.2   Protein content

Each purified antigen bulk should be tested for total protein content using a suitable method.

> The total protein content may be calculated from measurement of an earlier purification process intermediate.

A.5.1.3   Antigen content

The antigen content should be measured on the purified antigen bulk or the adsorbed antigen bulk (see section A.6.3.7) using an appropriate method.

The ratio of antigen content to protein content may be calculated and monitored for each purified antigen bulk.

International standards and reference reagents are not available for the control of hepatitis E vaccine antigen content. Therefore, product-specific reference preparations should be developed and used.

A.5.1.4   Sterility tests for bacteria and fungi

Each purified antigen bulk should be tested for bacterial and fungal sterility, as specified in Part A, section 5.2 of the WHO General requirements for the sterility of biological substances (*73*), or by a method approved by the NRA. Alternatively, this test can be performed on the related adsorbed antigen bulks if the purified bulk is not stored prior to adsorption.

WHO Technical Report Series, No. 1016, 2019

A.5.1.5 Percentage of intact monomer

The integrity of the HEV protein should be carefully monitored at least in the early stages of process validation and should be assessed by suitable methods. The purity assay (see section A.5.1.1) may also serve to assess the integrity of the HEV protein monomer. This test could be omitted, subject to the agreement of the NRA.

A.5.1.6 Particle size and morphology

The protein is expected to form particles of heterogeneous size; the size and morphology of the particles should be assessed and monitored. The distribution of particle sizes should be determined as a parameter of process control. This test may be omitted once consistency of production has been established, with the agreement of the NRA.

> Suitable methods for assessing particle size include dynamic light scattering, size-exclusion chromatography–high-performance liquid chromatography (SEC–HPLC) and transmission electron microscopy (TEM). A reference preparation should be included for comparison.

A.5.1.7 Tests for reagents used during purification or other phases of manufacture

A test should be carried out to detect the presence of any potentially hazardous reagents used during manufacture, using a method(s) approved by the NRA. This test may be omitted upon demonstration that the process consistently eliminates the reagent from the purified antigen bulks, subject to the agreement of the NRA.

A.5.1.8 Tests for residual host-derived material

Where a eukaryotic expression system is used, the amount of residual host-cell DNA derived from the expression system should be determined in each purified antigen bulk using suitably sensitive methods. The level of host-cell DNA should not exceed the maximum level agreed with the NRA, taking into consideration issues such as those discussed in the WHO Recommendations for the evaluation of animal cell cultures as substrates for the manufacture of biological medicinal products and for the characterization of cell banks (7).

These tests may be omitted upon demonstration that the process consistently inactivates the biological activity of the residual DNA or reduces the amount and size of the contaminating residual DNA present in the purified antigen bulks, subject to the agreement of the NRA.

Levels of residual protein from the host cell should be determined for all expression systems.

A.5.1.9 Test for viral clearance

When an insect or mammalian cell substrate is used for the production of antigens, the production process should be validated in terms of its capacity to remove and/or inactivate adventitious viruses – as described in the Q5A guidelines of the International Council for Harmonisation of Technical Requirements for Pharmaceuticals for Human Use (*75*). This testing is performed during vaccine manufacturing development or as part of process validation.

If a replicating viral vector such as a baculovirus is used, the production process should be validated for its capacity to eliminate (by removal and/or inactivation) residual recombinant virus.

A.6 Control of adsorbed antigen bulk

In cases where the adsorbed antigen bulk is further modified by dilution or addition of excipients to generate the final bulk, the considerations described below apply. Where the adsorbed bulk is filled directly without further modification it is the final bulk and this section does not apply (see instead section A.7).

A.6.1 Addition of adjuvant

The purified HEV antigen may be adsorbed onto an adjuvant such as an aluminium salt or other substance. Both the adjuvant and the concentration used should be approved by the NRA.

A.6.2 Storage

Until the adjuvanted antigen bulk is formulated into the final bulk, the suspension should be stored under conditions shown by the manufacturer to allow it to retain the desired biological activity. Hold times should be approved by the NRA.

A.6.3 Tests on adsorbed antigen bulk

All tests and specifications for adsorbed antigen bulk, unless otherwise specified, should be approved by the NRA.

A.6.3.1 Sterility tests for bacteria and fungi

Each adsorbed antigen bulk should be tested for bacterial and fungal sterility, as specified in Part A, section 5.2 of the WHO General requirements for the sterility of biological substances (*73*), or using a method approved by the NRA.

A.6.3.2 Bacterial endotoxins

Each adsorbed antigen bulk should be tested for bacterial endotoxins using a method approved by the NRA.

If it is inappropriate to test the adsorbed antigen bulk, the test should be performed on the purified antigen bulk prior to adsorption, subject to the agreement of the NRA.

A.6.3.3   Identity

Each adsorbed antigen bulk should be identified as the appropriate HEV antigen using a suitable method. The test for antigen content may also serve as the identity test. This test may be omitted if it is performed on the finished product.

A.6.3.4   Adjuvant concentration

Adsorbed antigen bulk should be assayed for adjuvant content.

A.6.3.5   Degree of adsorption

The degree of adsorption (completeness of adsorption) of the antigen to the adjuvant should be assessed, if applicable.

This test may be omitted upon demonstration of process consistency, subject to the agreement of the NRA.

A.6.3.6   pH

The pH value of the adsorbed antigen bulk should be monitored until production consistency is demonstrated, subject to the agreement of the NRA.

A.6.3.7   Antigen content

The antigen content of the adsorbed antigen bulk should be measured using appropriate methods. If this test is conducted on the purified antigen bulk, it may be omitted from the testing of the adsorbed antigen bulk.

International standards and reference reagents are not available for the control of hepatitis E vaccine antigen content. Therefore, product-specific reference preparations should be developed and used.

A.7   Control of final bulk

The antigen concentration in the final formulation should be sufficient to ensure that the dose is consistent with that shown to be safe and effective in human clinical trials. Should an adjuvant be added to the vaccine formulation, the adjuvant and the concentration used should be approved by the NRA.

The operations necessary for preparing the final bulk should be conducted in such a way as to avoid contamination of the product. In preparing the final bulk vaccine, any substances that are added to the product (such as diluents, stabilizers or adjuvants) should have been shown to the satisfaction of the NRA not to impair the safety and efficacy of the vaccine at the concentration used.

The final bulk should be stored under conditions shown by the manufacturer to allow it to retain the desired biological activity until it is filled into containers.

A.7.1   Tests on the final bulk

All tests and specifications for the final bulk should be approved by the NRA, unless otherwise specified. Where the antigen bulk is the final formulation, the tests below will be performed in accordance with section A.6 above at the level of the adsorbed antigen bulk and not repeated here.

A.7.1.1   Sterility tests for bacteria and fungi

Each final bulk should be tested for bacterial and fungal sterility, as specified in Part A, section 5.2 of the WHO General requirements for the sterility of biological substances (*73*), or using a method approved by the NRA.

A.7.1.2   Adjuvant content

Each final bulk should be assayed for adjuvant content.

Where aluminium compounds are used, the aluminium content should not exceed 1.25 mg per single human vaccine dose.

Tests for adjuvant content on the final bulk may be omitted if conducted on each final lot derived from the final bulk.

A.7.1.3   Degree of adsorption

The degree of adsorption (completeness of adsorption) of the antigen to the adjuvant in each final bulk should be assessed, if applicable, (for example, if the adjuvant is aluminium salts).

This test may be omitted upon demonstration of process consistency subject to the agreement of the NRA, or if performed on the final lot.

A.7.1.4   Preservative content

The final bulk should be tested for the presence of preservative, if added. The method used and the permitted concentration should be approved by the NRA.

A.7.1.5   Potency

The potency of each formulated final bulk before filling should be assessed by an appropriate in vivo method. If an in vivo potency test is used to test final fill lots, this test may be omitted on the formulated final bulk before filling. The methods used for antibody detection in the in vivo test and for the analysis of data should be approved by the NRA. The vaccine potency should be compared with that of a reference preparation approved by the NRA.

In vitro methods such as ELISA may be developed to assess potency. With the approval of the NRA, the in vitro assay may replace the in vivo assay when appropriately validated and when consistency of production is demonstrated.

Manufacturers should establish a product-specific reference preparation that is traceable to a specific lot of vaccine, or to bulks used in the production of a specific lot, which has been shown to be efficacious in clinical trials. The performance of this reference vaccine should be monitored by trend analysis using relevant test parameters and the reference vaccine should be replaced when necessary. An established procedure for replacing reference vaccines should be in place (*76, 77*).

A.7.1.6 Osmolality

The osmolality of the final bulk should be tested. The osmolality test may be omitted if performed on the final lot.

> An alternative test (for example, freezing point) may be used as a surrogate measure for ionic strength/osmolality.

A.8 Filling and containers

The requirements concerning filling and containers given in WHO good manufacturing practices for pharmaceutical products: main principles (*68*) and WHO good manufacturing practices for biological products (*69*) should apply to vaccine filled in the final form.

Care should be taken to ensure that the materials of which the container and, if applicable, the transference devices and closure are made do not adversely affect the quality of the vaccine.

Manufacturers should provide the NRA with adequate data to prove the stability of the product under appropriate conditions of storage and shipping.

A.9 Control tests on the final filled lot

The following tests should be performed on each final filled lot (that is, in the final containers). Unless otherwise justified and authorized, the tests should be performed on labelled containers from each final filled lot by means of validated methods approved by the NRA. All tests and specifications, including methods used and permitted concentrations, should be approved by the NRA, unless otherwise specified.

A.9.1 Inspection of containers

Every container in each final lot should be inspected visually or mechanically, and those showing abnormalities (for example, improper sealing, clumping or presence of particles) should be discarded and recorded for each relevant abnormality. A limit should be established for the percentage of containers rejected to trigger investigation of the cause, potentially resulting in batch failure.

A.9.2 Appearance

The appearance of the vaccine should be described with respect to its form and colour.

A.9.3 Identity

An identity test should be performed on at least one container from each final lot, using a validated method approved by the NRA. The potency test may serve as the identity test.

A.9.4 Sterility tests for bacteria and fungi

Each final lot should be tested for bacterial and fungal sterility, as specified in Part A, section 5.2 of the WHO General requirements for the sterility of biological substances (*73*), or using a method approved by the NRA.

A.9.5 pH and osmolality

The pH value and osmolality of the final lot should be tested. The osmolality test may be omitted if performed on the final bulk. The osmolality test may also be omitted for routine lot release upon demonstration of product consistency, subject to the agreement of the NRA.

> An alternative test (for example, freezing point) may be used as a surrogate measure for ionic strength/osmolality.

A.9.6 Preservatives

Each final lot should be tested for the presence of preservative, if added.

A.9.7 Test for pyrogenic substances

Each final lot should be tested for pyrogenic substances. Where appropriate, tests for endotoxin – for example, the limulus amoebocyte lysate (LAL) test – should be performed. However, where there is interference in the test (for example, from the adjuvant) a test for pyrogens in rabbits should be performed.

> A suitably validated monocyte-activation test may also be considered as an alternative to the rabbit pyrogen test.

> The test is conducted until consistency of production is demonstrated, subject to the agreement of the NRA.

A.9.8 Adjuvant content

Each final lot should be assayed for adjuvant content, if applicable. Where aluminium compounds are used, the aluminium content should not exceed 1.25 mg per single human vaccine dose.

A.9.9 Extractable volume

For vaccines filled into single-dose containers, the extractable content should be checked and shown to be not less than the intended dose.

For vaccines filled into multi-dose containers, the extractable content should be checked and should be shown to be sufficient for the intended number of doses.

A.9.10 Degree of adsorption

The degree of adsorption to the adjuvant (completeness of adsorption) of each antigen present in each final vaccine lot should be assessed, if applicable, and the limit should be approved by the NRA.

This test may be omitted for routine lot release upon demonstration of product consistency, subject to the agreement of the NRA.

A.9.11 Potency

A potency test should be carried out on each final lot as outlined above in section A.7.1.5. However, if the in vivo potency test has been performed on the final formulated bulk, the test on the final lot may be omitted, subject to the agreement of the NRA.

A.10 Records

The requirements given in WHO good manufacturing practices for pharmaceutical products: main principles (68) and WHO good manufacturing practices for biological products (69) should apply.

A.11 Retained samples

The requirements given in WHO good manufacturing practices for pharmaceutical products: main principles (68) and WHO good manufacturing practices for biological products (69) should apply.

A.12 Labelling

The requirements given in WHO good manufacturing practices for pharmaceutical products: main principles (68) and WHO good manufacturing practices for biological products (69) should apply. In the case of recombinant hepatitis E vaccines, the label on the carton, the container or the leaflet accompanying the container should state:

- that the vaccine has been prepared from recombinant bacterial cells, or another expression system;
- the genotype of the HEV antigen present in the preparation;
- the protein/antigen content and potency per dose;
- the number of doses, if the product is issued in a multi-dose container;
- the name and maximum quantity of any residual antibiotic present in the vaccine;
- the name and concentration of any preservative added;
- the name and concentration of any adjuvant added;
- the name and concentration of any other excipient added;
- the temperature recommended during storage and transport;
- the expiry date;
- the name of the manufacturer;
- the lot/batch number; and
- any special dosing schedules.

A.13 Distribution and transport

The requirements given in WHO good manufacturing practices for pharmaceutical products: main principles (68) and WHO good manufacturing practices for biological products (69) should apply. Further guidance is provided in the WHO Model guidance for the storage and transport of time- and temperature-sensitive pharmaceutical products (78).

A.14 Stability testing, storage and expiry date

A.14.1 Stability testing

Adequate stability studies form an essential part of vaccine development. Current guidance on the evaluation of vaccine stability is provided in the WHO Guidelines on stability evaluation of vaccines (79). Stability testing should be performed at different stages of production – namely on single antigen harvests or single harvest pools, purified antigen bulk, final bulk (whenever materials are stored before further processing) and final lot. Stability-indicating parameters appropriate to the stage of production should be defined or selected. A shelf-life should be assigned to all in-process materials during vaccine production –

WHO Technical Report Series, No. 1016, 2019

particularly intermediates such as single antigen harvests, purified antigen bulk and final bulk.

The stability and expiry date of the vaccine in its final container, maintained at the recommended storage temperature up to the expiry date, should be demonstrated to the satisfaction of the NRA using final containers from at least three final lots made from different purified antigen bulks.

Accelerated stability tests may be undertaken to provide additional information on the overall characteristics of a vaccine and may also aid in assessing comparability should the manufacturer decide to change aspects of manufacturing.

The formulation of vaccine antigens and adjuvant (if used) must be stable throughout the shelf-life of the vaccine. Acceptable limits for stability should be agreed with the NRA. Following licensure, ongoing monitoring of vaccine stability is recommended to support shelf-life specifications and to refine the stability profile (*79*). Data should be provided to the NRA in accordance with local regulatory requirements.

The final stability-testing programme should be approved by the NRA and should include an agreed set of stability-indicating parameters, procedures for the ongoing collection and sharing of stability data, and criteria for rejecting vaccines.

A.14.2 Storage conditions

The final lot should be kept at 2–8 °C. If other storage conditions are used they should be fully validated and approved by the NRA. The storage conditions used should ensure that the minimum vaccine potency specified on the label of the container or package will be maintained after release and until the end of the shelf-life, provided that the vaccine is stored under the recommended conditions. During storage, adsorbed vaccines should not be frozen.

If a vaccine has been shown to be stable at temperature ranges higher than the approved 2–8 °C range, it may be stored under extended controlled temperature conditions for a defined period, subject to the agreement of the NRA (*80*).

A.14.3 Expiry date

The expiry date should be based on the shelf-life supported by stability studies and should be approved by the NRA. The expiry date should be based on the date of blending of final bulk, the date of filling or the date of the first valid potency test on the final lot.

Where an in vivo potency test is used, the date of the potency test is the date on which the test animals are inoculated.

Part B. Nonclinical evaluation of recombinant hepatitis E vaccines

The nonclinical evaluation of hepatitis E vaccines should be based on the WHO guidelines on nonclinical evaluation of vaccines (5) which provide details on the design, conduct, analysis and evaluation of nonclinical studies. Further guidance on the general principles for the nonclinical evaluation of vaccine adjuvants and adjuvanted vaccines can be found in separate WHO guidelines (8).

Prior to the clinical testing of any new hepatitis E vaccine in humans there should be extensive product characterization, proof-of-concept studies, immunogenicity studies and safety testing in animals. The extent of nonclinical evaluation will depend on the complexity of the vaccine formulation on a case-by-case basis. The following specific issues should be considered in the context of the development of recombinant hepatitis E vaccines based on the ORF2-encoded viral capsid protein.

B.1 Strategy for cloning and expressing the gene product

The HEV genome contains three open reading frames. Of these, ORF2 codes for the viral capsid protein which is the target of neutralizing antibodies against HEV (*81–83*).

A full description should be given of the biological characteristics of the host cell and expression vectors used in production. This should include details of: (a) the construction, genetics and structure of the expression vector; (b) the origin and identification of the gene that is being cloned; and (c) potential adventitious retrovirus-like particles (and/or their genetic markers) in mammalian cell-based expression systems. The physiological measures used to promote and control the expression of the cloned gene in the host cell should also be described in detail.

Data should be provided to demonstrate the genetic stability of the expression system beyond the passage level used for production. Any instability of the expression system occurring in the seed culture or after a production-scale run (for example, involving rearrangements, deletions or insertions of nucleotides) must be documented. NRA approval should be obtained for the system used.

B.2 Product characterization and process development

Rigorous identification and characterization of recombinant DNA-derived vaccines is required as part of the application for marketing authorization. The ways in which these products differ chemically, structurally, biologically or immunologically from the naturally occurring antigen must be fully documented. Such differences could arise during processing at the genetic or post-translational level, or during purification.

The expressed protein should be characterized by biochemical, biophysical and immunological methods such as SDS-PAGE, isoelectric focusing, circular dichroism, matrix-assisted laser desorption/ionization time-of-flight mass spectrometry (MALDI-TOF), N-terminal sequencing, high-performance size-exclusion chromatography (HPSEC) and binding activity to monoclonal antibodies. The immunogenicity of the protein should be analysed in an appropriate animal model.

It is crucially important that vaccine production processes are appropriately standardized and controlled to ensure consistency in manufacturing, and in the collection of nonclinical data that may indicate potency and safety in humans. The extent of product characterization may vary according to the stage of development. The vaccine lots used in nonclinical studies should be adequately representative of the formulation intended for use in clinical investigation and, ideally, should be the same lots as those used in clinical trials. If this is not feasible, the lots used in nonclinical studies should be comparable to clinical lots with respect to physicochemical characteristics, stability and formulation.

B.3 Pharmacodynamic studies

B.3.1 Immunogenicity studies

The immunogenicity of the vaccine should be evaluated in relevant animal species that respond well to the vaccine antigen (for example, rodent, rabbit, swine or non-human primate) (84). Immunogenicity data can provide initial insights into the immunological characteristics of the vaccine antigen and are useful in evaluating the vaccine formulation and underlying protective mechanisms, and in justifying the inclusion of an adjuvant.

Nonclinical passive immunization studies in non-human primates and human epidemiology studies indicate that humoral immunity is probably the primary effector mechanism that directly mediates protection against HEV. Indeed, clear correlation between serum IgG responses to vaccine antigen and protection has been demonstrated in clinical (85) and nonclinical (86) studies of recombinant hepatitis E capsid-based vaccines. On this basis, it is recommended that the evaluation of vaccine immunogenicity should include an assessment of serum anti-HEV IgG antibodies.

Immunogenicity studies should establish a dose–response relationship by testing different doses of vaccine antigen. Ideally, immune responses are assessed after each dose of vaccine in line with the intended posology. For an adjuvanted vaccine, the advantage conferred by the adjuvant should be demonstrated on the basis of serological data – with or without additional elucidation of cellular immune response depending upon the adjuvant used.

B.3.2 Challenge studies

The protective effect of vaccine antigen should be evaluated in an appropriate animal model. Examples of animal models that are known to be experimentally permissive to infection by human HEV include swine (genotypes 3 and 4), rabbit (genotype 4), and different species of non-human primates such as cynomolgus macaques (genotypes 1 and 2) and rhesus macaques (genotypes 1–4) (*84*). Challenge studies conducted in non-human primates have demonstrated the protective immunity of hepatitis E vaccines which have subsequently been shown to be efficacious in humans (*62, 85*).

The animals used should be HEV-naive. The naive status of animals at baseline should be confirmed by the absence of detectable anti-HEV total IgG antibody in sera and absence of detectable HEV RNA in faeces and in sera. The virus used for animal challenge studies should correspond to the wild-type virus strain from which the vaccine antigen is derived.

The design of challenge studies may vary, depending on the platforms used to produce the vaccine. The vaccination of animals is usually conducted in accordance with the intended posology, with the subsequent challenge made when vaccinated animals develop peak protective responses. In general, challenge via the intravenous route is acceptable as transmission through the oral route is less efficacious. The challenge dose should be sufficiently high to ensure the establishment of reliable infection and/or histopathological hepatitis. Important end-points used to define protection should be specified in the study protocol and should include:

- infection marker such as HEV RNA in stool and serum at serial time points; and/or
- histopathological evidence of hepatitis using liver biopsy; and
- biochemical parameter of alanine aminotransferase (ALT) change at serial time points.

In addition, passive immunization studies in animal models that involve the transfer of antisera from human vaccinees to naive animals followed by HEV challenge might be useful in estimating a specific IgG titre associated with protection.

B.3.3 Cross-neutralization protection against different genotypes

The genetic differentiation of HEV strains is based on whether the nucleic acid variation of ORF2 between two viruses is more than 20%. According to this criterion, human HEV isolates are classified into four genotypes (genotypes 1–4). These four genotypes share a single serotype based on their immunoreactivity and cross-neutralization (*87, 88*). Therefore, hepatitis E vaccine based on recombinant

ORF2 derived from a given genotype is expected to provide protection against all four HEV genotypes. Results from preclinical and clinical studies have substantiated this expectation. In preclinical animal models the same protection was observed in animals challenged with different genotypes of HEV following immunization with recombinant ORF2 protein derived from a single genotype. For example, Purcell et al. (*89*) and Li et al. (*61*) demonstrated that immunization with recombinant ORF2 protein derived from genotype 1 HEV was able to protect against genotype 1, 2, 3 and 4 HEV infection in non-human primate models. In addition, a vaccine based on recombinant ORF2 protein derived from genotype 4 HEV provided cross-protection against genotypes 1 and 4 HEV infection in a non-human primate model (*90*). Studies conducted in an HEV rabbit model have indicated that recombinant capsid proteins derived from genotype 1 HEV cross-protects against genotype 4 HEV infection (*91, 92*).

Furthermore, during clinical trials conducted in China and Nepal, a recombinant ORF2 protein vaccine derived from genotype 1 HEV sequences was found to protect against acute hepatitis caused by genotypes 1 and 4 HEV infection (*63, 85, 92*).

Based on biochemical analysis of the recombinant capsid proteins, a cross-genotype and neutralizing epitope (as recognized by monoclonal antibody 8G12) was identified in both genotypes 1 and 4 HEV (*93*). The monoclonal antibody 8G12 was shown to block the binding of naturally acquired antibodies in human and animal sera. The presence of these "8G12-like" antibodies or the epitopes recognized by these antibodies could be regarded as a partial demonstration of cross-genotype protection elicited by vaccines based on antigens derived from a given type.

To date, only limited data on cross-protection are available from completed clinical trials with recombinant HEV capsid-based vaccines. If cross-protection against heterologous viruses is claimed then challenge studies should be conducted in appropriate animal models to evaluate the potential for such cross-protection.

B.4   Biodistribution studies

Pharmacokinetic studies are not required for recombinant human hepatitis E vaccines. If a novel excipient (including a novel adjuvant) is included in the vaccine then a biodistribution study should be considered (*8*).

B.5   Toxicology studies

Toxicology studies should be undertaken in accordance with the WHO guidelines on nonclinical evaluation of vaccines (*5*). Such studies should be performed using the final vaccine formulation in relevant animal species and should reflect the intended clinical use of the vaccine (5). Repeated-dose toxicity and local tolerance should be evaluated in relevant species following good laboratory practice (GLP) principles, prior to the initiation of early human clinical trials. Because the target population for hepatitis E vaccines includes women of childbearing age, GLP-compliant reproductive and developmental toxicity studies are also required.

In general, toxicity evaluation in one relevant species is justified. The route and dosing regimen used should reflect the intended clinical use. For the evaluation of developmental toxicity, the dosing regimen should consider one or two doses prior to mating so that pregnant animals, embryos and fetuses are exposed to a maximal vaccine response during the critical window of organogenesis.

If the vaccine is formulated with a novel adjuvant, nonclinical toxicology studies should be conducted as appropriate for the adjuvant concerned, and the recommendations provided in the WHO Guidelines on the nonclinical evaluation of vaccine adjuvants and adjuvanted vaccines should be followed (8).

If a novel cell substrate (that is, a substrate that has not been previously licensed or used in humans) is used for the production of a hepatitis E vaccine, safety aspects (such as potential immune responses elicited by residual host-cell proteins) should be investigated in a suitable animal model. Such studies should be undertaken particularly if the final product contains an adjuvant that might enhance responses to low levels of residual proteins.

Part C. Clinical evaluation of recombinant hepatitis E vaccines

C.1 Introduction

Clinical trials should adhere to the principles described in the WHO Guidelines for good clinical practice (GCP) for trials on pharmaceutical products (94). General guidance on vaccine clinical development programmes is provided in the WHO Guidelines on clinical evaluation of vaccines: regulatory expectations (6) and is not repeated here. This section addresses issues for clinical development programmes that are specific to, or of special concern for, vaccines intended to prevent clinically apparent infections with HEV.

C.2 Assays

This section considers:

- serological assays for establishing the baseline serostatus of trial subjects and evaluating the humoral immune response to vaccination (see also section C.3); and

WHO Technical Report Series, No. 1016, 2019

- serological and virus detection assays for laboratory confirmation of acute hepatitis caused by HEV infection in vaccine efficacy trials (see also section C.4).

Sponsors should also consult section 5.3.3 of the WHO Guidelines on clinical evaluation of vaccines: regulatory expectations (*6*).

C.2.1 Serological assays

C.2.1.1 Functional antibody

Currently there is no well-established assay for measuring anti-HEV neutralizing antibody. Since there is no efficient HEV cell infection model, a direct measurement of anti-HEV neutralizing antibody is not feasible. Neutralizing antibody has been estimated using methods such as real-time PCR (*95*) or an immunofluorescence foci assay (IFA) to detect virus, but these methods are not standardized or suitable for processing large numbers of sera and each has its drawbacks. Sponsors are encouraged to develop high-throughput assays for anti-HEV neutralizing antibody. For example, a potential high-throughput neutralization assay based on recombinant HEV capsid particles has been compared with IFA and with the measurement of anti-HEV IgG using sera from HEV-infected and vaccinated macaques (*95*).

C.2.1.2 Total binding antibody

For the purposes of estimating the immune response to vaccination, sponsors may choose to develop in-house anti-HEV IgG assays in which the antigen used to coat the wells is the same as – or at least a truncated version of – that used in the vaccine. It is recommended that the quantitation of anti-HEV IgG should be referenced to the WHO standard sera (*96*) as part of the validation of the assay. Using the selected assay methodology, a cut-off value should be identified and justified for distinguishing seronegative and seropositive sera.

For the detection of acute infection with HEV, commercial assays are available for detecting HEV-specific IgG, IgM, IgA and total immunoglobulin. These commercial assays vary considerably in their use of synthetic or recombinant antigen, viral strain origin and genotype, viral gene product(s) and detection method – for example, anti-HEV IgM antibody detection commonly uses a μ chain capture ELISA whereas IgG antibody detection usually involves a direct antigen-coating ELISA with secondary enzyme conjugated antibody. Comparative studies have shown considerable differences in the sensitivity and specificity of commercially available assays, with even more variability for IgM compared to IgG assays (*52, 53*). The assays used to detect and quantify anti-HEV antibody in suspected cases of hepatitis E in efficacy trials must be adequately justified, taking into account what is known about their performance characteristics.

C.2.2 Virus detection assays

Appropriate HEV RNA or antigen detection assays are required to confirm the presence of the virus in blood and/or stools of suspected cases of hepatitis E (see section C.4). Commercial quantitative PCR assays are available along with WHO HEV RNA international reference preparations for genotype 3a and 3b strains (66, 67, 97). Assays with different targets (for example, assays that target ORF2 or the ORF2/3 overlapping region) have been shown to have different performance characteristics. The ability of assays to detect and quantify HEV RNA from specific genotypes should be taken into account when selecting the method to be used in trials.

In vaccine efficacy trials it is recommended that HEV should be identified at least to genotype level for all PCR-positive cases. The fragments that are amplified by real-time PCR are usually less than 100 nucleotides in length and are located on conserved parts of the genome. Therefore, additional genomic sequencing (which published data suggest may be targeted to a specific region) is currently required to determine the HEV (sub-)genotype. Sponsors should provide full details of the methodology applied and appropriate controls should be used.

C.3 Immunogenicity

C.3.1 Formulation, dose and regimen

C.3.1.1 Primary series

Hepatitis E vaccines will be used mainly or exclusively in regions with relatively high rates of clinically apparent infections. However, pre-vaccination testing for HEV serostatus will not be feasible in routine use. In naturally primed individuals (not all of whom may have detectable pre-vaccination anti-HEV IgG) the first dose of hepatitis E vaccine may elicit large increments in antibody due to an anamnestic response. In contrast, multiple doses of the same vaccine may be required to achieve similar antibody levels in HEV-naive subjects. Consequently, it is important that the primary series should be selected on the basis of the immune responses observed in subjects who are seronegative – including seronegative subjects who are unlikely to have been naturally primed.

In the absence of an established immune correlate of protection for HEV, the selection of the vaccine dose and regimen may be based on reaching an antibody plateau response unless this is precluded by concerns over reactogenicity. It is desirable that immunogenicity studies should explore the minimum number of doses and the shortest dose interval(s) required to achieve a plateau immune response.

<h3>C.3.1.2   Need for revaccination</h3>

In the absence of an immune correlate of protection, it is recommended that the possible need for revaccination is not based solely upon waning antibody levels. There should be planned long-term follow-up for hepatitis E cases in vaccine efficacy trials, and/or data should be collected from vaccine effectiveness studies to determine waning protection against clinically apparent HEV infection (see section C.4.2.7).

In anticipation that revaccination may be necessary to maintain protection, it is recommended that the immune response to additional doses of vaccine is assessed. For example, subjects enrolled into an immunogenicity trial could be sub-randomized to receive further doses at predefined intervals after completion of a primary series. The immune response to additional doses could be compared with the post-primary response of the same individuals and/or compared with the response to a single dose administered to previously unvaccinated and seronegative control subjects.

<h3>C.3.1.3   Cross-protection</h3>

The ability of a candidate hepatitis E vaccine to protect against a range of wild-type strains covering the four main HEV genotypes may vary according to the vaccine construct. It is important that this should be investigated in nonclinical studies (see section B.3.3).

In clinical trials in which vaccine-elicited antibody is determined against the antigen in the vaccine (see section C.2.1.2), it is recommended that IgG is also measured using antigens derived from a range of wild-type HEVs. If marked differences are observed in IgG antibody when measured using vaccine versus non-vaccine antigens and/or by HEV genotype, it would be of particular interest to assess whether a similar effect is observed for functional antibody levels. In addition, depending on the range of investigations already completed, it may be appropriate to conduct additional nonclinical studies to evaluate the possible implications of the findings for protection before proceeding to the conducting of efficacy trials.

<h3>C.3.2   Special populations</h3>

Thus far, the efficacy of hepatitis E vaccination has been demonstrated in healthy subjects aged 16 years and above – most of whom have been under 45 years of age. There may be interest in the use of hepatitis E vaccines in younger age groups and/or subjects at particular risk of developing severe or fulminant hepatitis (for example, during pregnancy and in individuals with pre-existing liver disease) and/or immunodeficient subjects who are at risk of developing chronic HEV infection. If a vaccine has already been shown to be efficacious in healthy adults it may be possible, on the basis of safety and immunogenicity data, to extend its use to various special populations. For example:

- There may be interest in completing primary vaccination before the period of greatest risk – in which case, safety and immunogenicity data should be generated to support the use of appropriate regimen(s) in specific paediatric age subgroups.

- Section 5.6.4.2 of the WHO Guidelines on clinical evaluation of vaccines: regulatory expectations (6) discusses the evaluation of vaccine safety and immunogenicity during pregnancy. Protection against hepatitis E disease by vaccination during pregnancy (as opposed to the vaccination of women before or between pregnancies) would require the development of a vaccine that could elicit antibody levels that are likely to be protective (for example, similar to those observed in adults enrolled in vaccine efficacy trials) after a single dose or after two doses administered within a short interval.

- Subjects with pre-existing liver disease and immunodeficient subjects may have very variable immune responses to vaccination depending on the underlying cause and specific nature of their condition. Vaccine regimens should be supported by immune responses documented in specific subgroups that are representative of the intended target populations.

C.4 Efficacy

C.4.1 Requirement for a demonstration of vaccine efficacy

It is currently recommended that the protective efficacy of a candidate vaccine against clinically apparent HEV infection should be evaluated in a pre-licensure vaccine efficacy trial. The following considerations apply:

- At the time of preparing these WHO Recommendations there is one vaccine against hepatitis E that is licensed in one country (See General considerations) (62, 63).

- This licensed vaccine is not widely used and it is not included in national immunization programmes. As a result, the use of a control group that does not receive vaccination against hepatitis E is possible.

- In jurisdictions in which a licensed vaccine is available, it is possible that individual NRAs may consider that licensure can be based on a trial that evaluates the efficacy of the candidate vaccine relative to that of the licensed vaccine in a population similar to that in which the efficacy of the licensed vaccine was established.

- The lack of an immune correlate of protection against hepatitis E does not rule out immunobridging a candidate vaccine to a licensed vaccine that has been shown to be efficacious. However, this approach is possible only if both vaccines contain the same antigen(s) so that immune responses can be compared directly. In addition, the demonstration of efficacy of the first licensed vaccine was confined to HEV genotypes 1 and 4 and it is not known whether the protective immune response may vary between genotypes. Furthermore, the baseline seropositivity rate of the population in which efficacy was demonstrated was estimated at 47% (based on data from less than one tenth of the total subjects randomized into the trial) (63). It cannot be assumed that the point estimate of vaccine efficacy would be applicable to populations with very different pre-vaccination seropositivity rates.

Taking these considerations into account, the focus of this section is on clinical development programmes that include vaccine efficacy trials in which the control group does not receive vaccination against hepatitis E. Most of the recommendations are also applicable to trials in which the control group receives a licensed vaccine against hepatitis E. Clinical programmes leading to licensure based on immunobridging are not addressed in this guidance. The general principles to consider are discussed in sections 5.6.2 and 6.3.3 of the WHO Guidelines on clinical evaluation of vaccines: regulatory expectations (6).

C.4.2 Considerations for efficacy trial design

C.4.2.1 Primary objective

The primary objective will be to demonstrate that the candidate vaccine protects against clinically apparent (that is, symptomatic) HEV infection caused by any genotype (see section C.4.2.4).

- It is not required for efficacy to be shown against asymptomatic HEV infection. With the exception of immunodeficient subjects (who may develop chronic infection with possible sequelae) asymptomatic infection is of no clinical significance.
- It is not required for vaccine efficacy trials to be powered to demonstrate genotype-specific efficacy (see section C.4.2.2).

C.4.2.2 Trial sites

Efficacy trials will be conducted in endemic areas in which the estimated attack rate for clinically apparent HEV infection is sufficient to complete enrolment into an adequately powered vaccine efficacy trial within a reasonable time frame. Sites may be chosen on the basis of available public health disease-surveillance data and/or pre-trial evaluations of epidemiology conducted by the sponsor. In two prior efficacy trials (*62–64, 85*), HEV genotypes that caused clinically apparent infections in the control (placebo) groups were limited to strains circulating at the trial sites in the years in which they were conducted. Sponsors are encouraged to consider selecting sites in a range of geographical areas in which different genotypes are circulating and/or to conduct separate vaccine efficacy trials in regions with different genotype distributions.

C.4.2.3 Subject selection criteria

Because of the peak age incidence of hepatitis E it is likely that vaccine efficacy trials will target adolescents and adults. An upper age limit may be set depending on the age-specific attack rates.

In endemic areas, the adult population will include a variable proportion of subjects who are seropositive for IgG against HEV. Options for subject selection include the following:

- Adults could be enrolled without knowledge of their baseline serostatus for HEV – which is the usual approach in vaccine efficacy trials conducted in endemic regions. This provides an assessment of the benefit of vaccination over and above the level of pre-existing protection against HEV infection due to natural exposure. The proportion of subjects enrolled who are seropositive at the time of enrolment should be estimated retrospectively by determining anti-HEV IgG in samples obtained from all, or a randomly selected subset of, subjects prior to vaccination. This information is helpful when considering extrapolation of the estimate of vaccine efficacy observed to other regions not included in the trial.

- A possible alternative approach would be to pre-screen subjects for anti-HEV IgG and to enrol only those considered to be seronegative on the basis of a threshold determined by the assay used. This may allow for a smaller sample size to be randomized into the trial due to an expected higher attack rate; however, it is also possible that seronegative adults are less likely to encounter HEV compared to seropositive adults of a similar age range and resident in the same region due to differences in their living conditions. Therefore, detailed knowledge of the local epidemiology of hepatitis E should be taken into account before choosing this approach.

C.4.2.4 Primary end-point

In accordance with the recommended primary objective, the primary end-point should be clinically apparent acute hepatitis that is confirmed to be due to HEV.

Sponsors could consider appointing an independent data-adjudication committee to review the data and determine which subjects meet the case definition to be counted in the primary analysis.

C.4.2.4.1 *Clinical features for the case definition*

The clinical features that trigger subjects to present to study site staff or to a local designated health-care facility for laboratory investigations for acute hepatitis E should be selected with the aim of capturing as many cases as possible while limiting unnecessary investigations. On this basis it is reasonable to define a possible case of acute viral hepatitis requiring laboratory investigation as an illness presenting with any, or a minimum number of, signs and symptoms – including malaise, fatigue, anorexia, right upper quadrant tenderness for longer than 3 days or any duration of jaundice or dark urine. Additional symptoms that could be considered include any abdominal pain, nausea or vomiting that persists for at least 3 days and for which there is no known likely explanation.

C.4.2.4.2 *Laboratory confirmation of acute hepatitis E infection*

It is recommended that the laboratory confirmation of acute hepatitis E cases should be conducted in a designated central laboratory. If more than one central laboratory is necessary for practical reasons, it is essential that the laboratories use identical methodologies, and consideration should be given to testing a randomly selected subset of samples at each laboratory to assess concordance.

There is variability in the onset and duration of elevated ALT levels in serum, detectable HEV RNA in serum or stool, the appearance of anti-HEV IgM and the appearance of (or detectable increase in) anti-HEV IgG in relation to the first appearance of symptoms. An increase in ALT to at least 2.5-fold the upper limit of normal (ULN) based on the local or central laboratory normal range should lead to investigations to determine whether HEV is the causative agent. If the first sample does not show a ≥ 2.5-fold elevation in ALT, the test should be repeated after approximately 1–2 weeks for any subject with jaundice, persistent symptoms or elevated total serum bilirubin in the first sample.

The confirmation of HEV as causative of the clinical picture should be based on any two or more of the following:

- IgM against HEV – which is often detectable at the time of onset of clinical symptoms but may peak after 1–2 weeks, and in some cases remains detectable for several months;
- at least a 4-fold rise in anti-HEV IgG between the first sample and a convalescent sample;
- detection of HEV RNA in blood or in stool – which is usually short-lived but which may persist for longer in stool than in blood.

To avoid cases being missed, protocols should plan for appropriately timed repeat specimens to be collected (for example, at 2–6 weeks after the first sample) from individuals with elevated ALT. Since HEV RNA is most likely to be detectable early in the course of a clinical illness, it is recommended that samples are obtained as early as possible and, if negative, that repeat testing is conducted after a short interval.

Samples obtained at first presentation should also be tested to detect acute infection with HEV or coinfection with other hepatitis viruses that can cause the same clinical picture, including testing for:

- IgM against hepatitis A virus
- hepatitis B virus surface antigen and anti-core IgM
- antibody against hepatitis C virus and/or hepatitis C virus RNA.

If the first sample is negative for evidence of acute infection with hepatitis A, B, C or E viruses and further samples are indicated to rule out hepatitis E, it is recommended that these should also be retested for evidence of hepatitis A, B and C viruses to document any possible coinfections.

C.4.2.5 Primary, secondary and other analyses

In a vaccine efficacy trial, it may be permissible that the primary analysis includes only confirmed acute hepatitis E cases – whether there is evidence of coinfection with other hepatitis viruses or not – as follows:

- in subjects who completed the vaccination series within predetermined visit windows, if more than one dose is required; and
- with symptom onset occurring more than a defined period after the only or final dose of the series that takes into account what is known about the timing of the post-dose anti-HEV IgG peak.

This approach gives the most optimistic estimation of vaccine efficacy.

If the primary analysis is confined to cases counted as described above it is essential that predefined secondary analyses are carried out to estimate vaccine efficacy based on confirmed cases of clinically apparent HEV infection defined and counted as follows:

- all cases in subjects who received at least one assigned dose as randomized and regardless of adherence to study visit windows;
- cases that occurred at any time after the last dose received (that is, counted from the day of dosing) in those who completed the assigned number of doses;
- cases that occurred after each sequential dose, depending on the number of doses in the series and counted from the day of dosing.

Vaccine efficacy should be explored according to HEV genotype if this is feasible, depending on the numbers of cases that occur due to individual genotypes.

It is recommended that an additional analysis should explore any differences in clinical or laboratory features (including severity) between cases that occur in the candidate vaccine group and the control group (whether the control group receives placebo or a licensed vaccine against hepatitis E). The analysis should take into account whether the severity observed in individual subjects could reflect coinfection with other hepatitis viruses – whether acute (most likely coinfection with hepatitis A) or chronic (that is, acute hepatitis E occurring in subjects who have chronic hepatitis B or C infection).

C.4.2.6 Case ascertainment

It is recommended that an active case-ascertainment strategy is used throughout the time frame of a vaccine efficacy trial. This is essential at least up to the time of the primary analysis, which may be conducted after a specific number of total cases has been accumulated or after a predefined period in which a sufficient number of cases are expected to occur to estimate vaccine efficacy.

C.4.2.7 Duration of protection

While the primary analysis may lead to licensure, it is recommended that trials continue to use active case ascertainment to follow up subjects for several years to provide data on waning vaccine protection without unblinding of treatment assignment at the level of the individual. These data can be reported at some time after licensure of the vaccine and may point to the need for further doses to be administered at intervals to maintain protection.

C.4.2.8 Vaccine effectiveness

The need for vaccine effectiveness studies should be established at the time of licensure.

If longer-term follow-up within a pre-licensure trial is not considered to be feasible, the duration of vaccine protection should be investigated within a vaccine effectiveness study and/or as part of routine disease surveillance conducted by public health authorities. Furthermore, the efficacy of the vaccine against individual genotypes should be explored as part of a vaccine effectiveness study and/or during routine disease surveillance.

C.5 Safety

Evaluation of the safety of candidate hepatitis E vaccines should be undertaken in accordance with the recommendations made in section 7 of the WHO Guidelines on clinical evaluation of vaccines: regulatory expectations (6). If the primary series consists of several vaccine doses it is important to document whether reactogenicity increases with sequential doses. Additionally, the safety of post-primary doses should be evaluated. There may be special considerations for vaccine safety depending on the vaccine construct and the intended target population (for example, if the vaccine is proposed for administration during pregnancy).

If a candidate vaccine is evaluated in a large pre-licensure trial, and if the safety profile documented during immunogenicity trials did not give rise to any major concerns, it may be acceptable for a full assessment of safety (that is, including detailed documentation of local and systemic reactogenicity, as well as all unsolicited adverse events) to be confined to a randomized subset of the total subjects. Serious adverse events should be documented in all subjects enrolled at all trial sites.

Part D. Recommendations for NRAs

D.1   General recommendations

The general recommendations for NRAs and NCLs given in the WHO Guidelines for national authorities on quality assurance for biological products (*98*) and WHO Guidelines for independent lot release of vaccines by regulatory authorities (*99*) should apply. These recommendations specify that no new biological substance should be released until consistency of lot manufacturing and quality has been demonstrated.

The detailed production and control procedures – as well as any significant changes in them that may affect the quality, safety and efficacy of recombinant hepatitis E vaccines – should be discussed with and approved by the NRA (*100*). For control purposes, the relevant international reference preparations currently in force should be obtained for the purpose of calibrating national, regional and working standards (*101*). The NRA may obtain from the manufacturer the product-specific or working reference to be used for lot release.

Consistency of production has been recognized as an essential component in the quality assurance of recombinant hepatitis E vaccines. In particular, the NRA should carefully monitor production records and quality control test results for clinical lots, as well as for a series of consecutive lots of the vaccine.

D.2   Official release and certification

A vaccine lot should be released only if it fulfils all national requirements and/or satisfies Part A of these WHO Recommendations (*99*).

A summary protocol for the manufacturing and control of recombinant hepatitis E vaccines, based on the model summary protocol provided in Appendix 1 and signed by the responsible official of the manufacturing

WHO Technical Report Series, No. 1016, 2019

establishment, should be prepared and submitted to the NRA in support of a request for the release of a vaccine for use.

A Lot Release Certificate signed by the appropriate NRA official should then be provided if requested by a manufacturing establishment and should certify whether or not the lot of vaccine in question meets all national requirements and/or Part A of these WHO Recommendations. The certificate should provide sufficient information on the vaccine lot. The purpose of this official national release certificate is to facilitate the exchange of vaccines between countries and should be provided to importers of the vaccines. A model NRA Lot Release Certificate is provided in Appendix 2.

Authors and acknowledgements

The first draft of these WHO Recommendations was prepared by a WHO drafting group comprising Dr E. Gurley, International Centre for Diarrheal Diseases Research, Bangladesh and Johns Hopkins University, the USA; Dr P. Minor, National Institute for Biological Standards and Control, the United Kingdom; Dr M. Powell, Medicines and Healthcare Products Regulatory Agency, the United Kingdom; Dr Y. Sun, Paul-Ehrlich-Institut, Germany; Dr R. Wagner, Paul-Ehrlich-Institut, Germany; Dr Y. Wang, National Institutes for Food and Drug Control, China; Dr Q. Zhao, Xiamen University, China; and Dr D. Lei, World Health Organization, Switzerland, taking into consideration the discussions and consensus reached during a WHO working group meeting to develop WHO recommendations to assure the quality, safety and efficacy of recombinant hepatitis E vaccines, held in Geneva, Switzerland, 11–12 May 2017 and attended by: Dr I. Ciglenecki, Médecins Sans Frontières International, Switzerland; Mr S. Gao, Xiamen Innovax Biotech Co. Ltd, China; Dr E. Gurley, International Centre for Diarrheal Diseases Research, Bangladesh and Johns Hopkins University, the USA; Mr B. Huang, Xiamen Innovax Biotech Co. Ltd, China; Dr N. Kamar, Toulouse University Hospital, France; Mrs D. Kusmiaty, National Quality Control Laboratory of Drug and Food, Indonesia; Dr P. Minor, National Institute for Biological Standards and Control, the United Kingdom; Dr M. Li, China Food and Drug Administration, China; Dr A. Lommel, Paul-Ehrlich-Institut, Germany; Dr J. Lynch, International Vaccine Institute, Republic of Korea; Dr K. Maithal, Zydus Cadila Healthcare Ltd, India; Dr C. Ngabéré, Ministry of Public Health, Chad; Dr S. Phumiamorn, Institute of Biological Products, Thailand; Dr M. Powell, Medicines and Healthcare Products Regulatory Agency, the United Kingdom; Dr H. Iftikhar Qureshi, Pakistan Health Research Council, Pakistan; Dr J.W.K. Shih, Xiamen Innovax Biotech Co. Ltd, China; Mr B. Shrestha, Walter Reed/AFRIMS Research Unit Nepal, Nepal; Dr D. Steele, Bill & Melinda Gates Foundation, the USA; Dr E. Teshale, Centers for Disease Control and Prevention, the USA; Dr R. Wagner, Paul-Ehrlich-Institut, Germany; Dr Y. Wang, National

Institutes for Food and Drug Control, China; Dr X. Wu, National Institutes for Food and Drug Control, China; Dr C. Young, Health Canada, Canada; Dr J. Zhang, Xiamen University, China; Dr Q. Zhao, Xiamen University, China; and Dr P. Duclos, Dr G. Enwere, Dr I. Knezevic, Dr O. Lapujade, Dr D. Lei and Ms C.A. Rodriguez-Hernandez, World Health Organization, Switzerland.

The resulting document was then posted on the WHO Biologicals website for a first round of public consultation from November 2017 to February 2018. A second draft was then prepared by Dr E. Gurley, Johns Hopkins Bloomberg School of Public Health, the USA; Dr P. Minor, Consultant, the United Kingdom; Dr M. Powell, Medicines and Healthcare Products Regulatory Agency, the United Kingdom; Dr Y. Sun, Paul-Ehrlich-Institut, Germany; Dr Q. Zhao, Xiamen University, China; Dr R. Wagner, Paul-Ehrlich-Institut, Germany; Dr Y. Wang, National Institutes for Food and Drug Control, China; and Dr D. Lei, World Health Organization, Switzerland, incorporating comments received from regulatory authorities, manufacturers and academia as appropriate.

A third draft was then prepared by Dr E. Gurley, Johns Hopkins Bloomberg School of Public Health, the USA; Dr P. Minor, Consultant, the United Kingdom; Dr M. Powell, Medicines and Healthcare Products Regulatory Agency, the United Kingdom; Dr Y. Sun, Paul-Ehrlich-Institut, Germany; Dr Y. Wang, National Institutes for Food and Drug Control, China; Dr Q. Zhao, Xiamen University, China; and Dr D. Lei World Health Organization, Switzerland, taking into consideration comments received during an informal consultation held in Beijing, China, 18–19 April 2018 and attended by: Dr E. Gurley, Johns Hopkins Bloomberg School of Public Health, the USA; Mr D. Minh Hung, Ministry of Health, Viet Nam; Dr M. Li, China Food and Drug Administration, China; Dr Z. Liang, National Institutes for Food and Drug Control, China; Dr J. Martin, National Institute for Biological Standards and Control, the United Kingdom; Dr P. Minor, Consultant, the United Kingdom; Dr C. Ngabéré, Ministry of Public Health, Chad; Dr S. Phumiamorn, Ministry of Public Health, Thailand; Dr H. Iftikhar Qureshi, Pakistan Health Research Council, Pakistan; Dr J. Shin, WHO Regional Office for the Western Pacific, Philippines; Mr Y. Tang, WHO Country Office, China; Mr B. Shrestha, Walter Reed/AFRIMS Research Unit Nepal, Nepal; Dr R. Simalango, National Agency of Drug and Food Control, Indonesia; Dr D. Steele, Bill & Melinda Gates Foundation, the USA; Dr Y. Sun, Paul-Ehrlich-Institut, Germany; Dr E. Teshale, Centers for Disease Control and Prevention, the USA; Dr Y. Wang, National Institutes for Food and Drug Control, China; Dr H. Wahu Triestano Wibowo, National Agency of Drug and Food Control, Indonesia; Dr X. Wu, National Institutes for Food and Drug Control, China; Dr M. Xu, National Institutes for Food and Drug Control, China; Dr X. Yao, China Food and Drug Administration, China; Dr J. Zhang, Xiamen University, China; Dr Q. Zhao, Xiamen University, China; and Dr D. Lei, World Health Organization, Switzerland; representatives from industry: Dr H. Chandra, Cadila

Healthcare Limited, Vaccine Technology Center, India; Ms W. Weidan Huang, Xiamen Innovax Biotech Co. Ltd, China; Dr B. Huang, Xiamen Innovax Biotech Co. Ltd, China; and Dr J.W.K. Shih, Xiamen Innovax Biotech Co. Ltd, China.

The resulting document was then posted on the WHO Biologicals website for a second round of public consultation from July to September 2018, and the document WHO/BS/2018.2348 was subsequently prepared by Dr D. Lei, Dr P. Minor, Dr M. Powell and Dr Y. Sun with contributions from other drafting group members and from Professor J. Zhang, Xiamen University, China, incorporating comments received from regulatory authorities, manufacturers and academia as appropriate.

Further changes were subsequently made to document WHO/BS/ 2018.2348 by the WHO Expert Committee on Biological Standardization.

References

1. Hepatitis E vaccine: WHO position paper, May 2015. Wkly Epidemiol Rec. No. 18, 1 May 2015; 90:185–200 (https://www.who.int/wer/2015/wer9018.pdf?ua=1, accessed 11 December 2018).

2. Safety profile of a recombinant hepatitis E vaccine. In: Global Advisory Committee on Vaccine Safety, 11–12 June 2014. Wkly Epidemiol Rec. No. 29, 18 July 2014;89:327–9 (https://www.who.int/vaccine_safety/committee/topics/hepatitise/Jun_2014/en/, accessed 11 December 2018).

3. Global health sector strategy on viral hepatitis 2016–2021. Towards ending viral hepatitis. Geneva: World Health Organization; 2016 (WHO/HIV/2016.06; http://apps.who.int/iris/bitstream/ 10665/246177/1/WHO-HIV-2016.06-eng.pdf, accessed 11 December 2018).

4. WHO informal consultation on WHO recommendations to assure the quality, safety and efficacy of recombinant hepatitis E vaccines. Beijing, China, 18–19 April 2018. Meeting report. Geneva: World Health Organization; 2018 (https://www.who.int/biologicals/areas/vaccines/hepatitis/ HEV_Recommendations_Report_of_Informal_Consultation_Beijing_11.19.2018.pdf?ua=1, accessed 26 January 2019).

5. WHO guidelines on nonclinical evaluation of vaccines. In: WHO Expert Committee on Biological Standardization: fifty-fourth report. Geneva: World Health Organization; 2005: Annex 1 (WHO Technical Report Series, No. 927; http://www.who.int/biologicals/publications/trs/areas/vaccines/ nonclinical_evaluation/ANNEX%201Nonclinical.P31-63.pdf?ua=1, accessed 11 December 2018).

6. Guidelines on clinical evaluation of vaccines: regulatory expectations. In: WHO Expert Committee on Biological Standardization: sixty-seventh report. Geneva: World Health Organization; 2017: Annex 9 (WHO Technical Report Series, No. 1004; http://www.who.int/entity/biologicals/expert_ committee/WHO_TRS_1004_web_Annex_9.pdf?ua=1, accessed 11 December 2018).

7. Recommendations for the evaluation of animal cell cultures as substrates for the manufacture of biological medicinal products and for the characterization of cell banks. In: WHO Expert Committee on Biological Standardization: sixty-first report. Geneva: World Health Organization; 2013: Annex 3 (WHO Technical Report Series, No. 978; http://www.who.int/biologicals/vaccines/ TRS_978_Annex_3.pdf?ua=1, accessed 11 December 2018).

8. Guidelines on the nonclinical evaluation of vaccine adjuvants and adjuvanted vaccines. In: WHO Expert Committee on Biological Standardization: sixty-fourth report. Geneva: World Health Organization; 2014: Annex 2 (WHO Technical Report Series, No. 987; http://www.who.int/ biologicals/areas/vaccines/TRS_987_Annex2.pdf?ua=1, accessed 11 December 2018).

9. Bradley DW. Hepatitis E virus: a brief review of the biology, molecular virology, and immunology of a novel virus. J Hepatol. 1995;22(1 Suppl):140–5 (abstract: https://www.ncbi.nlm.nih.gov/pubmed/7602068, accessed 11 December 2018).

10. Aggarwal R, Goel A. Advances in hepatitis E – I: virology, pathogenesis and diagnosis. Expert Rev Gastroenterol Hepatol. 2016;10(9):1053–63 (abstract: https://www.tandfonline.com/doi/abs/10.1080/17474124.2016.1185362?journalCode=ierh20, accessed 11 December 2018).

11. Sridhar S, Teng JLL, Chiu T-H, Lau SKP, Woo PCY. Hepatitis E virus genotypes and evolution: emergence of camel hepatitis E variants. Int J Mol Sci. 2017;18(4):869 (https://core.ac.uk/download/pdf/95560998.pdf, accessed 11 December 2018).

12. Smith DB, Simmonds P, International Committee on Taxonomy of Viruses Hepeviridae Study Group, Jameel S, Emerson SU, Harrison TJ, Meng X-J et al. Consensus proposals for classification of the family Hepeviridae. J Gen Virol. 2014;95(10):2223–32 (https://www.ncbi.nlm.nih.gov/pmc/articles/PMC4165930/, accessed 11 December 2018).

13. Zhang J, Shih JW, Wu T, Li S-W, Xia N-S. Development of the hepatitis E vaccine: from bench to field. Semin Liver Dis. 2013;33(1):79–88 (abstract: https://www.researchgate.net/publication/236129039_Development_of_the_Hepatitis_E_Vaccine_From_Bench_to_Field, accessed 11 December 2018).

14. Woo PCY, Lau SKP, Teng JLL, Cao K-Y, Wernery U, Schountz T et al. New hepatitis E virus genotype in Bactrian camels, Xinjiang, China, 2013. Emerg Infect Dis. 2016;22(12):2219–2221 (https://wwwnc.cdc.gov/eid/article/22/12/pdfs/16-0979.pdf, accessed 11 December 2018).

15. Teshale EH, Hu DJ. Hepatitis E: epidemiology and prevention. World J Hepatol. 2011;3(12):285–91 (https://www.ncbi.nlm.nih.gov/pmc/articles/PMC3246546/, accessed 11 December 2018).

16. Kamar N, Bendall R, Legrand-Abravanel F, Xia N-S, Ijaz S, Izopet J et al. Hepatitis E. Lancet. 2012;379(9835):2477–88 (abstract: https://www.thelancet.com/journals/lancet/article/PIIS0140-6736(11)61849-7/fulltext, accessed 11 December 2018).

17. The global prevalence of hepatitis E virus infection and susceptibility: a systematic review. Geneva: World Health Organization; 2010 (WHP/IVB/10.14; http://apps.who.int/iris/bitstream/handle/10665/70513/WHO_IVB_10.14_eng.pdf;sequence=1, accessed 11 December 2018).

18. Rein DB, Stevens GA, Theaker J, Wittenborn JS, Wiersma ST. The global burden of hepatitis E virus genotypes 1 and 2 in 2005. Hepatology. 2012;55(4):988–97 (https://aasldpubs.onlinelibrary.wiley.com/doi/pdf/10.1002/hep.25505, accessed 11 December 2018).

19. Matsuda H, Okada K, Takahashi K, Mishiro S. Severe hepatitis E virus infection after ingestion of uncooked liver from a wild boar. J Infect Dis. 2003;188(6):944 (https://academic.oup.com/jid/article/188/6/944/947999, accessed 11 December 2018).

20. Strategic Advisory Group of Experts on Immunization (SAGE), Hepatitis E Vaccine Working Group. Hepatitis E: epidemiology and disease burden. Geneva: World Health Organization; 2014 (http://www.who.int/immunization/sage/meetings/2014/october/1_HEV_burden_paper_final_03_Oct_14_yellow_book.pdf?ua=1, accessed 11 December 2018).

21. Kim J-H, Nelson KE, Panzner U, Kasture Y, Labrique AB, Wierzba TF. A systematic review of the epidemiology of hepatitis E virus in Africa. BMC Infect Dis. 2014;14:308 (https://www.ncbi.nlm.nih.gov/pmc/articles/PMC4055251/, accessed 11 December 2018). Erratum in BMC Infect Dis. 2017;17:187 (https://www.ncbi.nlm.nih.gov/pmc/articles/PMC5335775/, accessed 11 December 2018).

22. Buisson Y, Grandadam M, Nicand E, Cheval P, van Cuyck-Gandre H, Innis B et al. Identification of a novel hepatitis E virus in Nigeria. J Gen Virol. 2000;81(4):903–9 (https://www.researchgate.net/publication/12591347_Identification_of_a_novel_hepatitis_E_virus_in_Nigeria, accessed 11 December 2018).

23. Nicand E, Armstrong GL, Enouf V, Guthmann JP, Guerin J-P, Caron M et al. Genetic heterogeneity of hepatitis E virus in Darfur, Sudan, and neighboring Chad. J Med Virol. 2005;77(4):519–21 (http://fieldresearch.msf.org/msf/bitstream/10144/66016/1/342_hepatitis+darfur.pdf, accessed 12 December 2018).

24. Teshale EH, Grytdal SP, Howard C, Barry V, Kamili S, Drobeniuc J et al. Evidence of person-to-person transmission of hepatitis E virus during a large outbreak in Northern Uganda. Clin Infect Dis. 2010;50(7):1006–10 (https://academic.oup.com/cid/article/50/7/1006/318143, accessed 12 December 2018).

25. Teshale EH, Howard CM, Grytdal SP, Handzel TR, Barry V, Kamili S et al. Hepatitis E epidemic, Uganda. Emerg Infect Dis. 2010;16(1):126–9 (https://www.ncbi.nlm.nih.gov/pmc/articles/PMC2874362/, accessed 12 December 2018).

26. Thomson K, Dvorzak JL, Lagu J, Laku R, Dineen B, Schilperoord M et al. Investigation of hepatitis E outbreak among refugees – Upper Nile, South Sudan, 2012–2013. MMWR. 2013;62(29);581–6 (https://www.cdc.gov/mmwr/preview/mmwrhtml/mm6229a2.htm, accessed 12 December 2018).

27. Hepatitis E – Niger. Disease Outbreak News, 5 May 2017 [webpage]. Geneva: World Health Organization; 2017 (http://www.who.int/csr/don/05-may-2017-hepatitis-e-niger/en/, accessed 12 December 2018).

28. Sazzad HMS, Labrique AB, Teo C-G, Luby SP, Gurley ES. Surveillance at private laboratories identifies small outbreaks of hepatitis E in urban Bangladesh. Am J Trop Med Hyg. 2017; 96(2):395–9 (available at: http://www.ajtmh.org/content/journals/10.4269/ajtmh.16-0411, accessed 12 December 2018).

29. Hewitt PE, Ijaz S, Brailsford SR, Brett R, Dicks S, Haywood B et al. Hepatitis E virus in blood components: a prevalence and transmission study in southeast England. Lancet. 2014;384(9956): 1766–73 (https://www.thelancet.com/journals/lancet/article/PIIS0140-6736(14)61034-5/fulltext, accessed 12 December 2018).

30. Huzly D, Umhau M, Bettinger D, Cathomen T, Emmerich F, Hasselblatt P et al. Transfusion-transmitted hepatitis E in Germany, 2013. Euro Surveill. 2014;19(21):20812 (https://www.eurosurveillance.org/content/10.2807/1560-7917.ES2014.19.21.20812, accessed 12 December 2018).

31. Verghese VP, Robinson JL. A systematic review of hepatitis E virus infection in children. Clin Infect Dis. 2014;59(5):689–97 (https://academic.oup.com/cid/article/59/5/689/2895517, accessed 12 December 2018).

32. Viswanathan R. Infectious hepatitis in Delhi (1955–56): a critical study-epidemiology. Indian J Med Res. 1957;45(Suppl.1):1–29 (see: http://www.ijmr.org.in/, accessed 26 January 2019).

33. Tsarev SA, Tsareva TS, Emerson SU, Yarbough PO, Legters LJ, Moskal T et al. Infectivity titration of a prototype strain of hepatitis E virus in cynomolgus monkeys. J Med Virol. 1994;43(2): 135–42 (abstract: https://onlinelibrary.wiley.com/doi/pdf/10.1002/jmv.1890430207, accessed 12 December 2018).

34. Arora NK, Nanda SK, Gulati S, Ansari IH, Chawla MK, Gupta SD et al. Acute viral hepatitis types E, A, and B singly and in combination in acute liver failure in children in north India. J Med Virol. 1996;48(3):215–21 (abstract: https://onlinelibrary.wiley.com/doi/abs/10.1002/%28SICI%291096-9071%28199603%2948%3A3%3C215%3A%3AAID-JMV1%3E3.0.CO%3B2-B, accessed 12 December 2018).

35. Khuroo MS, Kamili S. Aetiology, clinical course and outcome of sporadic acute viral hepatitis in pregnancy. J Viral Hepat. 2003;10(1):61–9 (abstract: https://onlinelibrary.wiley.com/doi/abs/10.1046/j.1365-2893.2003.00398.x, accessed 12 December 2018).

36. Tsega E, Krawczynski K, Hansson BG, Nordenfelt E. Hepatitis E virus in pregnancy in Ethiopia. Ethiop Med J. 1993;31(3):173–81 (abstract: https://www.researchgate.net/publication/14794191_Hepatitis_E_virus_in_pregnancy_in_Ethiopia, accessed 12 December 2018).

37. Ramalingaswami V, Purcell RH. Waterborne non-A, non-B hepatitis. Lancet. 1988;331(8585):571–3 (abstract: https://www.thelancet.com/journals/lancet/article/PIIS0140-6736(88)91362-1/fulltext, accessed 12 December 2018).

38. Kumar A, Beniwal M, Kar P, Sharma JB, Murthy NS. Hepatitis E in pregnancy. Int J Gynaecol Obstet. 2004;85(3):240–4 (abstract: https://www.sciencedirect.com/science/article/pii/S0020729 203005241, accessed 12 December 2018).

39. Khuroo MS, Kamili S. Aetiology and prognostic factors in acute liver failure in India. J Viral Hepat. 2003;10(3):224–31 (abstract: https://onlinelibrary.wiley.com/doi/abs/10.1046/j.1365-2893. 2003.00415.x, accessed 12 December 2018).

40. Pérez-Gracia MT, Suay-García B, Mateos-Lindemann ML. Hepatitis E and pregnancy: current state. Rev Med Virol. 2017;27(3):e1929 (abstract: https://onlinelibrary.wiley.com/doi/abs/10.1002/rmv.1929, accessed 12 December 2018).

41. Navaneethan U, Al Mohajer M, Shata MT. Hepatitis E and pregnancy: understanding the pathogenesis. Liver Int. 2008;28(9):1190–9 (abstract: https://onlinelibrary.wiley.com/doi/full/10.1111/j.1478-3231.2008.01840.x, accessed 12 December 2018).

42. Kamar N, Selves J, Mansuy J-M, Ouezzani L, Péron J-M, Guitard J et al. Hepatitis E virus and chronic hepatitis in organ-transplant recipients. N Engl J Med. 2008;358(8):811–7 (https://www.nejm.org/doi/full/10.1056/NEJMoa0706992, accessed 12 December 2018).

43. Robbins A, Lambert D, Ehrhard F, Brodard V, Hentzien M, Lebrun D et al. Severe acute hepatitis E in an HIV infected patient: successful treatment with ribavirin. J Clin Virol. 2014;60(4): 422–3 (abstract: https://www.sciencedirect.com/science/article/pii/S1386653214001784, accessed 24 December 2018).

44. Fujiwara S, Yokokawa Y, Morino K, Hayasaka K, Kawabata M, Shimizu T. Chronic hepatitis E: a review of the literature. J Viral Hepat. 2014;21(2):78–89 (abstract: https://www.researchgate.net/publication/259565743_Chronic_hepatitis_E_A_review_of_the_literature, accessed 24 December 2018).

45. Crum-Cianflone NF, Curry J, Drobeniuc J, Weintrob A, Landrum M, Ganesan A et al. Hepatitis E virus infection in HIV-infected persons. Emerg Infect Dis. 2012;18(3):502–6 (https://www.ncbi.nlm.nih.gov/pmc/articles/PMC3309581/, accessed 24 December 2018).

46. Lee G-H, Tan B-H, Teo EC-Y, Lim S-G, Dan Y-Y, Wee A et al. Chronic infection with camelid hepatitis E virus in a liver transplant recipient who regularly consumes camel meat and milk. Gastroenterology. 2016;150(2):355–7 (https://www.gastrojournal.org/article/S0016-5085(15) 01585-1/fulltext, accessed 24 December 2018).

47. Khudyakov Y, Kamili S. Serological diagnostics of hepatitis E virus infection. Virus Res. 2011; 161(1):84–92 (abstract: https://www.sciencedirect.com/science/article/abs/pii/S016817021100 2292, accessed 24 December 2018).

48. Zhao C, Geng Y, Harrison TJ, Huang W, Song A, Wang Y. Evaluation of an antigen-capture EIA for the diagnosis of hepatitis E virus infection. J Viral Hepat. 2015;22(11):957–63 (abstract: https://onlinelibrary.wiley.com/doi/full/10.1111/jvh.12397, accessed 24 December 2018).

49. Bendall R, Ellis V, Ijaz S, Ali R, Dalton H. A comparison of two commercially available anti-HEV IgG kits and a re-evaluation of anti-HEV IgG seroprevalence data in developed countries. J Med Virol. 2010;82(5):799–805 (abstract: https://www.onlinelibrary.wiley.com/doi/abs/10.1002/jmv. 21656, accessed 24 December 2018).

50. Mansuy J-M, Bendall R, Legrand-Abravanel F, Sauné K, Miédouge M, Ellis V et al. Hepatitis E virus antibodies in blood donors, France. Emerg Infect Dis. 2011;17(12):2309–12 (https://www.ncbi.nlm.nih.gov/pmc/articles/PMC3311200/, accessed 24 December 2018).

51. Mansuy J-M, Legrand-Abravanel F, Calot J-P, Peron JM, Alric L, Agudo S et al. High prevalence of anti-hepatitis E virus antibodies in blood donors from south west France. J Med Virol. 2008; 80(2):289–93 (abstract: https://onlinelibrary.wiley.com/doi/abs/10.1002/jmv.21056, accessed 24 December 2018).

52. Vollmer T, Diekmann J, Eberhardt M, Knabbe C, Dreier J. Monitoring of anti-hepatitis E virus antibody seroconversion in asymptomatically infected blood donors: systematic comparison of nine commercial anti-HEV IgM and IgG assays. Viruses. 2016;8(8):232 (https://www.ncbi.nlm.nih.gov/pmc/articles/PMC4997594/, accessed 25 December 2018).

53. Sommerkorn FM, Schauer B, Schreiner T, Fickenscher H, Krumbholz A. Performance of hepatitis E virus (HEV)-antibody tests: a comparative analysis based on samples from individuals with direct contact to domestic pigs or wild boar in Germany. Med Microbiol Immunol. 2017;206(3):277–86 (abstract: https://link.springer.com/article/10.1007/s00430-017-0503-4, accessed 25 December 2018).

54. Wen G-P, Tang Z-M, Yang F, Zhang K, Ji W-F, Cai W et al. A valuable antigen detection method for diagnosis of acute hepatitis E. J Clin Microbiol. 2015;53(3):782–8 (https://www.ncbi.nlm.nih.gov/pmc/articles/PMC4390668/, accessed 25 December 2018).

55. Huang S, Zhang X, Jiang H, Yan Q, Ai X, Wang Y et al. Profile of acute infectious markers in sporadic hepatitis E. PLoS One. 2010;5(10):e13560 (https://www.ncbi.nlm.nih.gov/pmc/articles/PMC2958841/, accessed 25 December 2018).

56. Drobeniuc J, Meng J, Reuter G, Greene-Montfort T, Khudyakova N, Dimitrova Z et al. Serologic assays specific to immunoglobulin M antibodies against hepatitis E virus: pangenotypic evaluation of performances. Clin Infect Dis. 2010;51(3):e24–7 (https://academic.oup.com/cid/article/51/3/e24/310202, accessed 25 December 2018).

57. Kmush BL, Labrique AB, Dalton HR, Ahmed ZB, Ticehurst JR, Heaney CD et al. Two generations of "Gold Standards": the impact of a decade in hepatitis E virus testing innovation on population seroprevalence. Am J Trop Med Hyg. 2015;93(4):714–7 (https://www.ncbi.nlm.nih.gov/pmc/articles/PMC4596587/, accessed 25 December 2018).

58. Khuroo MS, Khuroo MS. Seroepidemiology of a second epidemic of hepatitis E in a population that had recorded first epidemic 30 years before and has been under surveillance since then. Hepatol Int. 2010;4(2):494–9 (https://www.ncbi.nlm.nih.gov/pmc/articles/PMC2900553/, accessed 25 December 2018). Erratum in Hepatol Int. 2010;4(2):536 (https://www.ncbi.nlm.nih.gov/pmc/articles/PMC2900555/, accessed 25 December 2018).

59. Su Y-Y, Huang S-J, Guo M, Zhao J, Yu H, He W-G et al. Persistence of antibodies acquired by natural hepatitis E virus infection and effects of vaccination. Clin Microbiol Infect. 2017;23(5):336.e1–4 (https://www.clinicalmicrobiologyandinfection.com/article/S1198-743X(16)30550-X/fulltext, accessed 25 December 2018).

60. Chadha MS, Walimbe AM, Arankalle VA. Retrospective serological analysis of hepatitis E patients: a long-term follow-up study. J Viral Hepat. 1999;6(6):457–61 (abstract: https://onlinelibrary.wiley.com/doi/abs/10.1046/j.1365-2893.1999.00190.x, accessed 25 December 2018).

61. Li SW, Zhang J, Li YM, Ou SH, Huang GY, He ZQ et al. A bacterially expressed particulate hepatitis E vaccine: antigenicity, immunogenicity and protectivity on primates. Vaccine. 2005;23(22):2893–901 (abstract: https://www.sciencedirect.com/science/article/pii/S0264410X0400920X, accessed 25 December 2018).

62. Zhang J, Liu C-B, Li R-C, Li Y-M, Zheng Y-J, Li Y-P et al. Randomized-controlled phase II clinical trial of a bacterially expressed recombinant hepatitis E vaccine. Vaccine. 2009;27(12):1869–74 (abstract: https://www.sciencedirect.com/science/article/pii/S0264410X09000061, accessed 25 December 2018).

63. Zhu F-C, Zhang J, Zhang X-F, Zhou C, Wang Z-Z, Huang S-J et al. Efficacy and safety of a recombinant hepatitis E vaccine in healthy adults: a large-scale, randomised, double-blind placebo-controlled, phase 3 trial. Lancet. 2010;376(9744):895–902 (abstract: https://www.thelancet.com/journals/lancet/article/PIIS0140-6736(10)61030-6/fulltext, accessed 25 December 2018).

64. Zhang J, Zhang X-F, Huang S-J, Wu T, Hu Y-M, Wang Z-Z et al. Long-term efficacy of a hepatitis E vaccine. N Engl J Med. 2015;372:914–22 (https://www.nejm.org/doi/full/10.1056/NEJMoa1406011, accessed 25 December 2018).

65. Collaborative study to assess the suitability of the proposed international standard for antibodies to hepatitis E virus. Prepared for the WHO Expert Committee on Biological Standardization, Geneva, 27–31 October 1997. Geneva: World Health Organization; 1997 (Document WHO/BS/97.1869).

66. Collaborative study to establish a World Health Organization international standard for hepatitis E virus RNA for nucleic acid amplification technology (NAT)-based assays. Prepared for the WHO Expert Committee on Biological Standardization, Geneva, 17–21 October 2011. Geneva: World Health Organization; 2011 (Document WHO/BS/2011.2175; http://apps.who.int/iris/bitstream/handle/10665/70783/WHO_BS_2011.2175_eng.pdf?sequence=1, accessed 25 December 2018).

67. Collaborative study to establish the 1st World Health Organization International Reference Panel for hepatitis E virus RNA genotypes for nucleic acid amplification technique (NAT)-based assays. Prepared for the WHO Expert Committee on Biological Standardization, Geneva, 12–16 October 2015. Geneva: World Health Organization; 2015. (Document WHO/BS/2015.2264; http://apps.who.int/iris/bitstream/handle/10665/197775/WHO_BS_2015.2264_eng.pdf?sequence=1&isAllowed=y, accessed 25 December 2018).

68. WHO good manufacturing practices for pharmaceutical products: main principles. In: WHO Expert Committee on Specifications for Pharmaceutical Preparations: forty-eighth report. Geneva: World Health Organization; 2014: Annex 2 (WHO Technical Report Series, No. 986; http://www.who.int/medicines/areas/quality_safety/quality_assurance/TRS986annex2.pdf?ua=1, accessed 25 December 2018).

69. WHO good manufacturing practices for biological products. In: WHO Expert Committee on Biological Standardization: sixty-sixth report. Geneva: World Health Organization; 2016: Annex 2 (WHO Technical Report Series, No. 999; http://www.who.int/biologicals/areas/vaccines/Annex_2_WHO_Good_manufacturing_practices_for_biological_products.pdf?ua=1, accessed 25 December 2018).

70. Derivation and characterisation of cell substrates used for production of biotechnological/biological products Q5D (Step 4). ICH Harmonised Tripartite Guideline. Geneva: International Conference on Harmonisation of Technical Requirements for Registration of Pharmaceuticals for Human Use; 1997 (http://www.ich.org/fileadmin/Public_Web_Site/ICH_Products/Guidelines/Quality/Q5D/Step4/Q5D_Guideline.pdf, accessed 25 December 2018).

71. Guidelines on the quality, safety and efficacy of biotherapeutic protein products prepared by recombinant DNA technology. In: WHO Expert Committee on Biological Standardization: sixty-fourth report. Geneva: World Health Organization; 2014: Annex 4 (WHO Technical Report Series, No. 987; http://www.who.int/biologicals/biotherapeutics/TRS_987_Annex4.pdf?ua=1, accessed 25 December 2018).

72. Recommendations to assure the quality, safety and efficacy of recombinant human papillomavirus virus-like particle vaccines. In: WHO Expert Committee on Biological Standardization: sixty-sixth report. Geneva: World Health Organization; 2016: Annex 4 (WHO Technical Report Series, No. 999; http://www.who.int/entity/biologicals/areas/vaccines/Annex_4_Recommendations_recombinant_human_papillomavirus_virus-like_particle_vaccines.pdf?ua=1, accessed 25 December 2018).

73. General requirements for the sterility of biological substances (Requirements for Biological Substances No. 6) (Revised 1973). In: WHO Expert Committee on Biological Standardization: twenty-fifth report. Geneva: World Health Organization; 1973: Annex 4 (WHO Technical Report Series, No. 530; http://www.who.int/biologicals/publications/trs/areas/vaccines/sterility/WHO_TRS_530_A4.pdf?ua=1, accessed 25 December 2018).

74. General requirements for the sterility of biological substances. (Requirements for Biological Substances No. 6, revised 1973, amendment 1995). In: WHO Expert Committee on Biological Standardization: forty-sixth report. Geneva: World Health Organization; 1998: Annex 3 (WHO Technical Report Series, No. 872; http://www.who.int/biologicals/publications/trs/areas/vaccines/sterility/WHO_TRS_872_A3.pdf, accessed 25 December 2018).

75. Quality of biotechnological products: viral safety evaluation of biotechnology products derived from cell lines of human or animal origin. ICH Topic Q5A (R1). (Step 5). ICH Harmonised Tripartite Guideline. London: European Medicines Agency; 2006 (Document CPMP/ICH/295/95; https://www.ema.europa.eu/documents/scientific-guideline/ich-q-5-r1-viral-safety-evaluation-biotechnology-products-derived-cell-lines-human-animal-origin_en.pdf, accessed 25 December 2018).

76. Recommendations to assure the quality, safety and efficacy of recombinant hepatitis B vaccines. In: WHO Expert Committee on Biological Standardization: sixty-first report. Geneva: World Health Organization; 2010: Annex 4 (WHO Technical Report Series, No. 978; http://www.who.int/biologicals/vaccines/TRS_978_Annex_4.pdf?ua=1, accessed 25 December 2018).

77. WHO manual for the establishment of national and other secondary standards for vaccines. Geneva: World Health Organization; 2011 (Document WHO/IVB/11.03; http://whqlibdoc.who.int/hq/2011/WHO_IVB_11.03_eng.pdf, accessed 25 December 2018).

78. Model guidance for the storage and transport of time- and temperature-sensitive pharmaceutical products. In: WHO Expert Committee on Specifications for Pharmaceutical Preparations: forty-fifth report. Geneva: World Health Organization; 2011: Annex 9 (WHO Technical Report Series, No. 961; http://www.who.int/medicines/areas/quality_safety/quality_assurance/ModelGuidanceForStorageTransportTRS961Annex9.pdf, accessed 25 December 2018).

79. Guidelines on stability evaluation of vaccines. In: WHO Expert Committee on Biological Standardization: fifty-seventh report. Geneva: World Health Organization; 2011: Annex 3 (WHO Technical Report Series, No. 962; http://www.who.int/biologicals/vaccines/Annex_3_WHO_TRS_962-3.pdf?ua=1, accessed 25 December 2018).

80. Guidelines on the stability evaluation of vaccines for use under extended controlled temperature conditions. In: WHO Expert Committee on Biological Standardization: sixty-sixth report. Geneva: World Health Organization; 2016: Annex 5 (WHO Technical Report Series, No. 999; http://www.who.int/biologicals/areas/vaccines/Annex_5_Guidelines_on_Stability_evaluation_vaccines_ECTC.pdf?ua=1, accessed 25 December 2018).

81. Zhang J, Gu Y, Ge SX, Li SW, He ZQ, Huang GY et al. Analysis of hepatitis E virus neutralization sites using monoclonal antibodies directed against a virus capsid protein. Vaccine. 2005; 23(22):2881–92 (abstract: https://www.sciencedirect.com/science/article/pii/S0264410X04009211, accessed 25 December 2018).

82. Schofield DJ, Glamann J, Emerson SU, Purcell RH. Identification by phage display and characterization of two neutralizing chimpanzee monoclonal antibodies to the hepatitis E virus capsid protein. J Virol. 2000;74(12):5548–55 (https://www.ncbi.nlm.nih.gov/pmc/articles/PMC112041/, accessed 25 December 2018).

83. Jun Z, Li S-W, Wu T, Zhao Q, Ng MH, Xia N-S. Hepatitis E virus: neutralizing sites, diagnosis, and protective immunity. Rev Med Virol. 2012;22(5):339–49 (abstract: https://www.researchgate.net/publication/225074114_Hepatitis_E_virus_Neutralizing_sites_diagnosis_and_protective_immunity, accessed 25 December 2018).

84. Yugo DM, Cossaboom CM, Meng X-J. Naturally occurring animal models of human hepatitis E virus infection. ILAR J. 2014;55(1):187–99 (https://academic.oup.com/ilarjournal/article/55/1/187/841499, accessed 11 January 2018).

85. Shrestha MP, Scott RM, Joshi DM, Mammen MP Jr, Thapa GB, Thapa N et al. Safety and efficacy of a recombinant hepatitis E vaccine. N Engl J Med. 2007;356(9):895–903 (https://www.nejm.org/doi/full/10.1056/NEJMoa061847, accessed 25 December 2018).

86. Tsarev SA, Tsareva TS, Emerson SU, Govindarajan S, Shapiro M, Gerin JL et al. Successful passive and active immunization of cynomolgus monkeys against hepatitis E. Proc Natl Acad Sci U S A. 1994;91(21):10198–202 (https://www.ncbi.nlm.nih.gov/pmc/articles/PMC44985/, accessed 25 December 2018).

87. Engle RE, Yu C, Emerson SU, Meng X-J, Purcell RH. Hepatitis E virus (HEV) capsid antigens derived from viruses of human and swine origin are equally efficient for detecting anti-HEV by enzyme immunoassay. J Clin Microbiol. 2002;40(12):4576–80 (https://www.ncbi.nlm.nih.gov/pmc/articles/PMC154628/, accessed 25 December 2018).

88. Meng J, Pillot J, Dai X, Fields HA, Khudyakov YE. Neutralization of different geographic strains of the hepatitis E virus with anti-hepatitis E virus-positive serum samples obtained from different sources. Virology. 1998;249:316–24 (https://core.ac.uk/download/pdf/82586903.pdf, accessed 25 December 2018).

89. Purcell RH, Nguyen H, Shapiro M, Engle RE, Govindarajan S, Blackwelder WC et al. Pre-clinical immunogenicity and efficacy trial of a recombinant hepatitis E vaccine. Vaccine. 2003;21(19–20):2607–15 (abstract: https://www.sciencedirect.com/science/article/pii/S0264410X03001002, accessed 25 December 2018).

90. Huang WJ, Zhang HY, Harrison TJ, Lan HY, Huang GY, Wang YC. Immunogenicity and protective efficacy in rhesus monkeys of a recombinant ORF2 protein from hepatitis E virus genotype 4. Arch Virol. 2009;154(3):481–8 (abstract: https://link.springer.com/article/10.1007%2Fs00705-009-0335-7, accessed 25 December 2018).

91. Liu P, Du Rj, Wang L, Han J, Liu L, Zhang Yl et al. Management of hepatitis E virus (HEV) zoonotic transmission: protection of rabbits against HEV challenge following immunization with HEV 239 vaccine. PLoS One. 2014;9(1):e87600 (https://www.ncbi.nlm.nih.gov/pmc/articles/PMC3907545/, accessed 25 December 2018).

92. Zhang Y, Zeng H, Liu P, Liu L, Xia J, Wang L et al. Hepatitis E vaccine immunization for rabbits to prevent animal HEV infection and zoonotic transmission. Vaccine. 2015;33(38):4922–8 (abstract: https://www.ncbi.nlm.nih.gov/pubmed/26212003, accessed 25 December 2018).

93. Gu Y, Tang X, Zhang X, Song C, Zheng M, Wang K et al. Structural basis for the neutralization of hepatitis E virus by a cross-genotype antibody. Cell Res. 2015;25(5):604–20 (https://www.ncbi.nlm.nih.gov/pmc/articles/PMC4423075/, accessed 25 December 2018).

94. Guidelines for good clinical practice (GCP) for trials on pharmaceutical products. In: WHO Expert Committee on the Use of Essential Drugs: sixth report. Geneva: World Health Organization; 1995: Annex 3 (WHO Technical Report Series, No. 850; http://apps.who.int/medicinedocs/pdf/whozip13e/whozip13e.pdf, accessed 14 January 2019).

95. Cai W, Tang Z-M, Wen G-P, Wang S-L, Ji W-F, Yang M et al. A high-throughput neutralizing assay for antibodies and sera against hepatitis E virus. Sci Rep. 2016;6:25141 (http://www.nature.com/articles/srep25141, accessed 25 December 2018).

96. Ferguson M, Walker D, Mast E, Fields H. Report of a collaborative study to assess the suitability of a reference reagent for antibodies to hepatitis E virus. Biologicals. 2002;30(1):43–8 (http://www.sciencedirect.com/science/article/pii/S104510560190315X, accessed 25 December 2018).

97. Baylis SA, Blümel J, Mizusawa S, Matsubayashi K, Sakata H, Okada Y et al. World Health Organization international standard to harmonize assays for detection of hepatitis E virus RNA. Emerg Infect Dis. 2013;19(5):729–35 (https://wwwnc.cdc.gov/eid/article/19/5/12-1845_article, accessed 25 December 2018).

98. Guidelines for national authorities on quality assurance for biological products. In: WHO Expert Committee on Biological Standardization: forty-second report. Geneva: World Health Organization; 1992: Annex 2 (WHO Technical Report Series, No. 822; http://www.who.int/biologicals/publications/trs/areas/biological_products/WHO_TRS_822_A2.pdf?ua=1, accessed 25 December 2018).

99. Guidelines for independent lot release of vaccines by regulatory authorities. In: WHO Expert Committee on Biological Standardization: sixty-first report. Geneva: World Health Organization; 2013: Annex 2 (WHO Technical Report Series, No. 978; http://www.who.int/biologicals/TRS_978_Annex_2.pdf?ua=1, accessed 25 December 2018).

100. Guidelines on procedures and data requirements for changes to approved vaccines. In: WHO Expert Committee on Biological Standardization: sixty-fifth report. Geneva: World Health Organization; 2015: Annex 4 (WHO Technical Report Series, 993; http://www.who.int/biologicals/vaccines/Annex4_Guidelines_changes_to_approved_vaccines_eng.pdf?ua=1, accessed 25 December 2018).

101. Recommendations for the preparation, characterization and establishment of international and other biological reference standards (revised 2004). In: WHO Expert Committee on Biological Standardization: fifty-fifth report. Geneva: World Health Organization; 2006: Annex 2 (WHO Technical Report Series, No. 932; http://www.who.int/immunization_standards/vaccine_reference_preparations/TRS932Annex%202_Inter%20_biol%20ef%20standards%20rev2004.pdf?ua=1, accessed 25 December 2018).

Appendix 1

Model summary protocol for the manufacturing and control of recombinant hepatitis E vaccines

The following summary protocol is intended for guidance. It indicates the information that should be provided as a minimum by the manufacturer to the NRA. Information and tests may be added or deleted/omitted as necessary with the approval of the NRA.

It is possible that a summary protocol for a specific product may differ in detail from the model provided. The essential point is that all relevant details demonstrating compliance with the licence and with the relevant WHO recommendations for a particular product should be provided in the protocol submitted.

The section concerning the final product must be accompanied by a sample of the label and a copy of the leaflet (package insert) that accompanies the vaccine container. If the protocol is being submitted in support of a request to permit importation, it must also be accompanied by a Lot Release Certificate from the NRA of the country in which the vaccine was produced or released, stating that the product meets national requirements as well as the recommendations in Part A of this document.

Summary information on final lot

International name: _______________________________________

Trade name/commercial name: _______________________________

Product licence (marketing authorization) number: ______________

Country: ____

Name and address of manufacturer: __________________________

Name and address of licence holder, if different: _______________

Final packaging lot number: ________________________________

Type of container: ____

Number of containers in this final lot: _______________________

Final container lot number: _________________________________

Date of manufacture: ______________________________________

Nature of final product (adsorbed): __________________________

Preservative and nominal concentration: ______________________

Volume of each single human dose: __________________________

Number of doses per final container: _________________________

Summary of the composition (include a summary of the qualitative and quantitative composition of the vaccine per human dose, including any adjuvant used and other excipients):

Shelf-life approved (months): _______________________

Expiry date: _______________________

Storage condition: _______________________

The following sections are intended for recording the results of the tests performed during the production of the vaccine, so that the complete document will provide evidence of consistency of production. If any test has to be repeated, this must be indicated. Any abnormal result must be recorded on a separate sheet.

Detailed information on manufacture and control

Starting materials

The information requested below is to be presented on each submission. Full details on master and working seed lots and cell banks are requested upon first submission only and whenever a change has been introduced.

Identity of seed lot strain used for
    vaccine production: _______________________

Reference number of seed lot: _______________________

Date(s) of reconstitution (or opening) of seed
    lot ampoule(s): _______________________

Single harvests used for preparing the bulk

Lot number(s): _______________________

Volume(s) of fermentation paste, storage temperature,
    storage time and approved storage period: _______________________

Name of the culture medium: _______________________

Date of inoculation: _______________________

Temperature of incubation: _______________________

Control of bacterial purity
    Method: _______________________

    Specification: _______________________

    Date: _______________________

    Result: _______________________

Date of harvest: _______________________________________

Volume of harvest: _______________________________________

Yield (mg/ml): _______________________________________

Volume after filtration: _______________________________________

Identity test
    Method: _______________________________________
    Specification: _______________________________________
    Date: _______________________________________
    Result: _______________________________________

Test for bacteria and fungi
    Method: _______________________________________
    Media: _______________________________________
    Volume inoculated: _______________________________________
    Date of start of test: _______________________________________
    Date of end of test: _______________________________________
    Result: _______________________________________

Test for Mycoplasmas (if applicable)
    Method: _______________________________________
    Volume inoculated: _______________________________________
    Date of start of test: _______________________________________
    Date of end of test: _______________________________________
    Result: _______________________________________

Test for adventitious agents (if applicable)
    Method: _______________________________________
    Specification: _______________________________________
    Date: _______________________________________
    Result: _______________________________________

Control of purified antigen bulk

Lot number of purified bulk: _______________________________________

Date of purification: _______________________________________

Volume(s), storage temperature, storage time
    and approved storage period: _______________________________________

Purity
    Method: _______________________________________
    Specification: _______________________________________

Date: ____

Result: ____

Protein content

Method: ____

Specification: ______________________________________

Date: ____

Result: ____

Antigen content

Method: ____

Specification: ______________________________________

Date: ____

Result: ____

Sterility test for bacteria and fungi

Method: ____

Media: ____

Volume inoculated: __________________________________

Date of start of test: _____________________________

Date of end of test: _______________________________

Result: ____

Percentage of intact monomer

Method: ____

Specification: ______________________________________

Date: ____

Result: ____

Particle size and morphology

Method: ____

Specification: ______________________________________

Date: ____

Result: ____

Test for reagents used during purification or other phases of manufacture (if relevant)

Method: ____

Specification: ______________________________________

Date: ____

Result: ____

Test for residual host-cell protein (if relevant)
    Method: ____
    Specification: ____________________________________
    Date: ____
    Result: ____

Test for residual host-cell DNA (if applicable)
    Method: ____
    Specification: ____________________________________
    Date: ____
    Result: ____

Test for viral clearance (if relevant)
    Method: ____
    Specification: ____________________________________
    Date: ____
    Result: ____

Control of adsorbed antigen bulk (if applicable)

Lot number of adsorbed antigen bulk: ________________________
Date of adsorption: ______________________________________
Volume(s), storage temperature, storage time
    and approved storage period: ____________________________

Sterility test for bacteria and fungi
    Method: ____
    Media: ____
    Volume inoculated: _______________________________
    Date of start of test: _____________________________
    Date of end of test: ______________________________
    Result: ____

Bacterial endotoxin
    Method: ____
    Specification: ____________________________________
    Date: ____
    Result: ____

Identity test
    Method: ____
    Specification: ____________________________________

Date: ____
Result: ____

Adjuvant content
 Method: ____
 Specification: ____
 Date: ____
 Result: ____

Degree of adsorption
 Method: ____
 Specification: ____
 Date: ____
 Result: ____

pH
 Method: ____
 Specification: ____
 Date: ____
 Result: ____

Antigen content
 Method: ____
 Specification: ____
 Date: ____
 Result: ____

Control of final bulk

Identification (lot number): ____

Date of manufacture/blending: ____

Volume(s), storage temperature, storage time
 and approved storage period ______________________________________

Blending:	Prescription (SHD)	Added
HEV antigen (mg):	______________	______________
Adjuvant:	______________	______________
Preservative (specify):	______________	______________
Others (salt):	______________	______________
Final volume (ml):	______________	______________

Sterility tests for bacteria and fungi
    Method: ____
    Media: ____
    Volume inoculated: ________________________________
    Date of start of test: _____________________________
    Date of end of test: ______________________________
    Result:

Adjuvant content
    Method: ____
    Specification: ____________________________________
    Date: ____
    Result: ____

Degree of adsorption
    Method: ____
    Specification: ____________________________________
    Date: ____
    Result: ____

Preservative content
    Method: ____
    Specification: ____________________________________
    Date: ____
    Result: ____

Potency test
In vivo assay (may be performed at final bulk stage)
    Species, strain, sex and weight specifications: ______________

    Number of mice tested: ____________________________
    Dates of vaccination, bleeding: ___________________
    Date of assay: ____________________________________
    Lot number of reference vaccine and
        assigned potency: ______________________________
    Vaccine doses (dilutions) and number of
        animals responding at each dose: ________________

    ED_{50} of reference and test vaccine: _______________
    Potency of test vaccine (with 95% fiducial limits): __________

If an in vitro assay is used

    Method: ____

    Specification: ____

    Date: ____

    Result: ____

Osmolality test

    Method: ____

    Specification: ____

    Date: ____

    Result: ____

Control of final lot

Lot number: ____

Date of filling: ____

Type of container: ____

Filling volume: ____

Number of containers after inspection: ________________________

Number and percentage of containers rejected: __________________

Appearance

    Method: ____

    Specification: ____

    Date: ____

    Result: ____

Identity test

    Method: ____

    Specification: ____

    Date: ____

    Result: ____

Sterility tests for bacteria and fungi

    Method: ____

    Media: ____

    Volume inoculated: _____________________________________

    Date of start of test: ____________________________________

    Date of end of test: ____________________________________

    Result: ____

Osmolality test

    Method: ____

    Specification: ____

    Date: ____

    Result: ____

pH

    Method: ____

    Specification: ____

    Date: ____

    Result: ____

Preservative content

    Method: ____

    Specification: ____

    Date: ____

    Result: ____

Test for pyrogenic substances

    Method: ____

    Specification: ____

    Date: ____

    Result: ____

Adjuvant content

    Method: ____

    Specification: ____

    Date: ____

    Result: ____

Extractable volume

    Method: ____

    Specification: ____

    Date: ____

    Result: ____

Degree of adsorption

    Method: ____

    Specification: ____

    Date: ____

    Result: ____

Potency test
In vivo assay (may be performed at final bulk stage)
    Species, strain, sex and weight specifications: _______________

    Number of mice tested: _______________
    Dates of vaccination, bleeding: _______________
    Date of assay: _______________
    Lot number of reference vaccine and
       assigned potency: _______________
    Vaccine doses (dilutions) and number of
       animals responding at each dose: _______________
    ED_{50} of reference and test vaccine: _______________
    Potency of test vaccine (with 95% fiducial limits): _______________

If an in vitro assay is used
    Method: _______________
    Lot number of reference and assigned potency: _______________
    Specification: _______________
    Date: _______________
    Result: _______________

Certification by the manufacturer

Name of Head of Quality Control (typed) _______________

Certification by the person from the control laboratory of the manufacturing company taking overall responsibility for the production and quality control of the vaccine.

I certify that lot no. _______________ of recombinant hepatitis E vaccine, whose number appears on the label of the final containers, meets all national requirements and/or satisfies Part A[1] of the WHO Recommendations to assure the quality, safety and efficacy of recombinant hepatitis E vaccines.[2]

Signature _______________
Name (typed) _______________
Date _______________

---

[1] With the exception of provisions on distribution and shipping, which the NRA may not be in a position to assess.
[2] WHO Technical Report Series, No. 1016, Annex 2.

Certification by the NRA

If the vaccine is to be exported, attach the NRA Lot Release Certificate (as shown in Appendix 2), a label from a final container and an instruction leaflet for users.

Appendix 2

Model NRA Lot Release Certificate for recombinant hepatitis E vaccines

Certificate no. _______________________

The following lot(s) of recombinant hepatitis E vaccine produced by _______________________ [1] in _______________________,[2] whose lot numbers appear on the labels of the final containers, meet all national requirements[3] and Part A[4] of the WHO Recommendations to assure the quality, safety and efficacy of recombinant hepatitis E vaccines[5] and comply with WHO good manufacturing practices for pharmaceutical products: main principles,[6] WHO good manufacturing practices for biological products[7] and Guidelines for independent lot release of vaccines by regulatory authorities.[8]

The release decision is based on _______________________ [9]

The certificate may include the following information:

- name and address of manufacturer;
- site(s) of manufacturing;
- trade name and common name of product;
- marketing authorization number;
- lot number(s) (including sub-lot numbers and packaging lot numbers if necessary);
- type of container used;
- number of doses per container;

---

[1] Name of manufacturer.

[2] Country of origin.

[3] If any national requirements have not been met, specify which one(s) and indicate why the release of the lot(s) has nevertheless been authorized by the NRA.

[4] With the exception of provisions on distribution and shipping, which the NRA may not be in a position to assess.

[5] WHO Technical Report Series, No. 1016, Annex 2.

[6] WHO Technical Report Series, No. 986, Annex 2.

[7] WHO Technical Report Series, No. 999, Annex 2.

[8] WHO Technical Report Series, No. 978, Annex 2.

[9] Evaluation of the summary protocol, independent laboratory testing and/or procedures specified in a defined document, and so on as appropriate.

- number of containers or lot size;
- date of start of period of validity (for example, manufacturing date) and expiry date;
- storage conditions;
- signature and function of the person authorized to issue the certificate;
- date of issue of certificate;
- certificate number.

The Director of the NRA (or other appropriate authority)

Name (typed) ____

Signature ____

Date ____

Annex 3

Guidelines for the safe development and production of vaccines to human pandemic influenza viruses and influenza viruses with pandemic potential

Replacement of Annex 5 of WHO Technical Report Series, No. 941; and the WHO 2009 A(H1N1) update; and the WHO 2013 A(H7N9) update

Guidelines published by the World Health Organization (WHO) are intended to be scientific and advisory in nature. Each of the following sections constitutes guidance for laboratories that test candidate influenza vaccine viruses, vaccine manufacturers and national regulatory authorities (NRAs). If an NRA so desires, these WHO Guidelines may be adopted as definitive national requirements, or modifications may be justified and made by the NRA. It is recommended that modifications to these Guidelines are made only on condition that such modifications ensure that the risks of introducing influenza viruses into the community are no greater than would be the case if these WHO Guidelines are followed.

Abbreviations

ABSL	biosafety level
CVV	candidate vaccine virus
EID_{50}	egg infectious dose 50%
FFP	filtering face-piece
GISRS	(WHO) Global Influenza Surveillance and Response System
GMP	good manufacturing practice(s)
HA	haemagglutinin
HEPA	high-efficiency particulate air
HPAI	highly pathogenic avian influenza
IVPI	intravenous pathogenicity index
IVPP	influenza virus(es) with pandemic potential
LAIV	live attenuated influenza vaccine
LPAI	low pathogenic avian influenza
MDCK	Madin-Darby Canine Kidney (cells)
NA	neuraminidase
NRA	national regulatory authority
OIE	World Organisation for Animal Health
PFU	plaque forming unit(s)
PPE	personal protective equipment
PR8	influenza A/Puerto Rico/8/34 virus (A/PR/8/34)
RG	reverse genetics
$TCID_{50}$	tissue culture infectious dose 50%

1. Introduction

Careful risk assessment and strict biosafety and biosecurity precautions are needed in laboratory and manufacturing environments in order to ensure the safe handling of human pandemic influenza viruses, candidate vaccine viruses (CVVs) and influenza viruses with pandemic potential (IVPP) as the uncontrolled release of such viruses could have a significant impact on public health. In 2007, the WHO biosafety risk assessment and guidelines for the production and quality control of human influenza pandemic vaccines were published (*1*) in response to the pandemic threat posed by highly pathogenic avian influenza (HPAI) A(H5N1) viruses and the need to begin vaccine development. Since the publication of this WHO guidance, experience in the use of both IVPP and pandemic influenza viruses in the development and production of CVVs has increased globally. This experience includes the development and testing of CVVs derived by reverse genetics (RG) from HPAI viruses – a development reflected in these revised WHO Guidelines. Moreover, in response to the 2009 pandemic caused by the A(H1N1)pdm09 subtype virus and the emergence of low pathogenic avian influenza (LPAI) A(H7N9) viruses that are able to infect humans and cause severe disease with a high case fatality rate, the 2007 guidance was updated on two occasions by WHO (*2, 3*). In addition, several WHO consultations – including the biannual WHO Vaccine Composition Meetings, the Global Action Plan for Influenza Vaccines (GAP) meetings and "switch" meetings[13] on influenza vaccine response at the start of a pandemic (*4–7*) – identified the testing timelines for CVVs as one of the bottlenecks to rapid vaccine responses. In light of these and other developments, requests were made to WHO by industry, regulators and laboratories of the WHO Global Influenza Surveillance and Response System (GISRS) to undertake a revision of the 2007 guidance.

In response, WHO convened a working group meeting on 9–10 May 2017 that was attended by experts, including representatives of WHO collaborating centres, WHO essential regulatory laboratories, national regulatory authorities (NRAs) for vaccine and biosafety regulation, manufacturers and the World Organisation for Animal Health (OIE). The working group reviewed cumulative experience, discussed the revision of the 2007 WHO guidance and reached a consensus on the outline and key elements of the revision (*8*). Subsequently, a draft revision was prepared and posted on the WHO website for public consultation. A WHO informal consultation was then held on 23–24 April 2018 to finalize the revision process (*9*). This document follows the risk assessment scheme used in the WHO biosafety guidance for pilot-lot vaccine

---

[13] Meetings relating to the issues involved in switching from seasonal influenza vaccine production to pandemic vaccine production in an emergency.

production (*10*). It also includes considerations relating to the greater scale of production needed to rapidly supply large quantities of vaccines, for which the risks are likely to be different to those for pilot lots. The document also takes into account the considerable experience gained from handling HPAI viruses and those classified as low virulence for avian species but highly virulent for humans.

2. Purpose and scope

These WHO Guidelines provide guidance to CVV-testing laboratories, vaccine manufacturers and NRAs on the safe development and production of human influenza vaccines in response to the threat of a pandemic. The document describes international biosafety expectations for pilot-scale and large-scale vaccine production and laboratory research. It is thus relevant to both vaccine development and vaccine manufacturing activities. It also specifies the measures to be taken to prevent or minimize the risk to workers involved in the development and production processes, and to prevent or minimize the risk of release of virus into the environment, including the risk of transmission to animals. Tests required to evaluate the safety of CVVs are also described. The document should be read in conjunction with the WHO *Laboratory biosafety manual* (*11*).

The guidance provided reflects greater knowledge of A(H5N1) subtype viruses (and other subtypes in general) and experience gained in the development and manufacture of vaccines against A(H5N1) viruses. Moreover, much has been learnt from experience with the A(H1N1)pdm09 virus, and from the production of vaccines against it. The guidance is also intended to apply to threats from any IVPP (for example, H2, H7 and H9 viruses) which may be virulent in humans. Manufacturers and laboratories handling HPAI viruses should consult their NRA to determine whether additional biosafety and biosecurity measures are required.

There is significant diversity in the pathogenicity of viruses used to make CVVs for the production of human vaccines and vaccines for other mammals. The transmission and pathogenicity of influenza viruses are multifactorial traits that are not completely understood (*12*). The haemagglutinin (HA) protein is the major virulence determinant of avian influenza viruses (*13*). Consequently, A(H5N1) HPAI viruses that cause fatal disease in humans have been used to produce reassortant viruses containing an HA that has been genetically modified to generate viruses of low pathogenicity for poultry. For viruses that are inherently less pathogenic for humans, the wild-type virus might be used directly for inactivated vaccine production (*14*). Thus, both reassortants derived by conventional reassortment and by RG – including those using synthetic nucleic acid as starting material (which may or may not be genetically modified) – and wild-type viruses are included in the scope of these Guidelines.

Although embryonated hens' eggs have traditionally been used to produce most influenza vaccines, cell culture techniques have also been successfully used for seasonal and pandemic vaccine production (*15, 16*). The guidance provided in this document applies to current vaccine production technologies using either eggs or cell culture.

These Guidelines also cover both inactivated vaccines and live attenuated influenza vaccines (LAIVs). To date, most efforts to develop CVVs for pandemic vaccines have been focused on the development of inactivated vaccine. However, seasonal LAIVs derived from the A/Ann Arbor/6/60 virus have been licensed in North America and Western Europe, while LAIVs derived from the A/Leningrad/134/17/57 virus have been licensed in China, India, the Russian Federation and Thailand (*17*).

Technologies not covered by these Guidelines include new generation technology platforms that do not use live influenza vaccine viruses for production (for example, expressed recombinant proteins, virus-like particles, DNA- and RNA-based vaccines and vectored vaccines) – though some general principles may be applicable.

The guidance provided on containment measures in this document applies to all facilities and laboratories that handle live influenza viruses, including not only the CVV and vaccine manufacturing facilities but also the quality control laboratories of vaccine manufacturers, national control laboratories and other specialist laboratories. The transport of live virus materials within and between these sites must comply with international and national specifications (*18*).

Finally, risk assessments for vaccine manufacture will vary according to whether production occurs during an interpandemic phase or during a pandemic alert phase or pandemic phase (*19*). These Guidelines emphasize the steps required to identify and minimize risks in vaccine manufacture during the interpandemic phase, while indicating modifications that may be appropriate in other phases. It should be noted that a pandemic preparedness approach covering both inactivated influenza vaccines and LAIVs (formerly called "mock-up pandemic vaccines") during the interpandemic phase has been accepted by the European Medicines Agency (EMA) (*20*).

3. Terminology

The definitions given below apply to the terms as used in these WHO Guidelines. These terms may have different meanings in other contexts.

Aerosol: a dispersion of solid or liquid particles of microscopic size in a gaseous medium.

Airlock: an area found at the entrances or exits of rooms that prevents air in one space from entering another space. Airlocks generally have two interlocked doors and a separate exhaust ventilation system. In some cases, a multiple-chamber airlock consisting of two or more airlocks joined together is used for additional control.

Backbone donor virus: an influenza virus that provides all or some non-glycoprotein internal genes to a reassortant virus. These genes may contain determinants of attenuation and/or confer high-growth/high-yield properties on the resulting reassortant virus.

Biosafety: the combination of physical and operational requirements and practices that protect personnel, the environment and the wider community against exposure to infectious materials during vaccine manufacture and quality control testing. Designation of laboratory facilities ranging from biosafety level (BSL) 1 to BSL4 and detailed principles for the operation of facilities at each level are set out in the WHO *Laboratory biosafety manual* (*11*) and in national or regional regulatory guidelines.

Biosafety committee: an institutional or organizational committee comprising individuals versed in the containment and handling of infectious materials.

Biosafety manual: a comprehensive document describing the physical and operational biosafety practices of the laboratory facility, with particular reference to infectious materials.

Biosafety officer: a staff member of an institution who has expertise in microbiology and infectious materials and who has responsibility for ensuring that the physical and operational practices required for the various levels of biosafety are carried out in accordance with the standard procedures of the institution.

Biosecurity: the protection and control of biological materials within laboratories and production facilities in order to prevent their unauthorized accessing, loss, theft, misuse, diversion or intentional release.

BSL2 or BSL3 enhanced: the use of additional physical and/or operational precautions, above those described for BSL2 or BSL3, based on a local risk assessment in consultation with the competent national authority and/or regulatory authority.

Bunded (area): an area that has either a permanent or a temporary barrier that is able to contain liquid and prevent leaks and spills from spreading contamination or damaging the facility (bunding).

Decontamination: a process by which influenza viruses are inactivated to prevent adverse health and/or environmental effects.

Egg infectious dose 50% (EID$_{50}$): the unit of infectious activity of a biological product or agent that causes infection in 50% of inoculated chicken embryos.

FFP2: a filtering face-piece (FFP) mask that provides high-level filtering capability against airborne transmissible microorganisms and generates an effective barrier to both droplets and fine aerosols to 94% efficiency.

FFP3: an FFP device (face-fitted mask) that provides high-level filtering capability against airborne transmissible microorganisms and generates an effective barrier to both droplets and fine aerosols to 99% efficiency (at 95 litres/ minute air flow).

Fumigation: the process whereby a gaseous chemical is applied to sterilize or disinfect surfaces in an enclosed space.

Good manufacturing practice(s) (GMP): that part of quality assurance which ensures that products are produced and controlled consistently to the quality standards appropriate to their intended use and as required by the marketing authorization.

High-efficiency particulate air (HEPA) filter: a filter capable of removing at least 99.97% of all airborne particles with a mean aerodynamic diameter of 0.3 μm (previously high-efficiency particulate absorber of various efficiencies).

Highly pathogenic avian influenza (HPAI) viruses: avian influenza viruses causing systemic infection and mortality in chickens which, to date, are limited to H5 and H7 subtypes containing a cleavage site in HA with multiple inserted amino acids (also referred to in the literature as a "multibasic" or "polybasic" cleavage site – though other insertions have also been identified). The designation HPAI does not refer to the virulence of these viruses in human or other mammalian hosts.

Inactivation: the process of rendering an influenza virus nonviable by application of heat, chemicals (for example, formalin or β-propiolactone), ultraviolet irradiation or other means.

Intravenous pathogenicity index (IVPI): an indicator used to classify an avian influenza virus as HPAI or LPAI on the basis of mortality and morbidity over a 10-day period following intravenous inoculation of chickens with the virus.

Low pathogenic avian influenza (LPAI) virus: avian influenza viruses causing infections in poultry leading to no disease, mild disease or moderate disease (see also **IVPI**). LPAI viruses typically contain an HA with a single basic amino acid preceding the site of proteolytic cleavage (also referred to as a "monobasic" cleavage site). The designation LPAI does not refer to the virulence of these viruses in human and other mammalian hosts.

N95: a respiratory protective device designed to achieve a very close facial fit and very efficient filtration of airborne particles. The designation N95 means that the respirator blocks at least 95% of very small (0.3 μm) test particles when fitted correctly.

Primary containment: a system of containment, usually a biological safety cabinet or closed container, which prevents the escape of a biological agent into the work environment.

Respirator hood: a respiratory protective device with an integral perimeter seal, valves and specialized filtration, used to protect the wearer from toxic fumes or particulates.

Risk assessment: a formalized and documented process for evaluating the potential risks that may be involved in a projected activity or undertaking.

Tissue culture infectious dose 50% (TCID$_{50}$): the unit of infectious activity of a biological product or agent that causes infection in 50% of inoculated tissue cultures.

Validation: the documented act of proving that any procedure, process, equipment, material, activity or system leads to the expected results.

4. Hazard identification

The hazards associated with vaccine manufacturing and laboratory testing of CVVs prepared from pandemic viruses and IVPP depend on: (a) the type of vaccine virus (reassortant or wild-type); (b) the method of production (egg-based, cell-culture-based or other); (c) whether it is an inactivated virus, live (attenuated) virus or recombinant virus-vectored vaccine; and (d) whether or not there are any deliberate modifications of the virus for attenuation or for enhanced immunogenicity and/or increased yield. Recombinant virus-vectored vaccines use replicating recombinant constructs based on viruses other than influenza virus (for example, modified vaccinia Ankara virus, adenovirus and vesicular stomatitis virus). The nature of their transgene, extent of virus shedding and the potential for recombination are outside the scope of the current document but are important factors that might need to be considered (*21, 22*).

4.1 Candidate vaccine viruses

CVVs for both LAIVs and inactivated influenza vaccines are generally produced through reassortment with well-defined backbone donor viruses – for example, human viruses A/Puerto Rico/8/34 (PR8), A/Ann Arbor/6/60 or A/Leningrad/134/17/57. Wild-type viruses may also be used for vaccine production if recommended by WHO and approved by the NRA. Furthermore, new backbone donor viruses for reassortment are being developed and evaluated to enhance vaccine yields and other desirable properties. Although it is likely that a high-growth reassortant will provide the basis for future pandemic vaccine development, it is conceivable that a wild-type virus could be used.

4.1.1 Reassortants

The genome of the influenza A virus is composed of eight individual single-stranded RNA segments of negative polarity. Segments 4 and 6 encode the two surface glycoproteins HA and neuraminidase (NA), respectively. HA is the major surface antigen of the virus, and antibodies directed against HA can protect from infection by neutralizing the virus. Antibodies to NA can inhibit viral infectivity at different points in the replication cycle and also have a role in protection from disease (*23*). The remaining six RNA segments ("internal protein genes") encode internal structural and nonstructural viral proteins. The segmented structure of the genome allows for the exchange (reassortment) of individual RNA segments between influenza viruses upon coinfection of a single cell with two or more influenza viruses.

The conventional method for reassortment involves preparing CVVs by the co-inoculation of embryonated hens' eggs or tissue culture with a WHO-recommended wild-type virus and a backbone donor virus with a high-growth (yield) or attenuated phenotype. Co-inoculation allows for the reassortment of genetic segments between the two viruses. Antiserum against the surface glycoproteins of the backbone donor virus is then used to select a reassortant CVV, which must contain the HA gene of the WHO-recommended vaccine virus (but which normally contains both the HA and NA genes of the WHO-recommended vaccine virus). Amplification in eggs (or cultured cells) results in positive selection for the optimal combination of internal genes providing a high-yield reassortant virus. Several weeks are usually required for the production, validation and antigenic analysis of the reassortant (*7*). The use of a CVV in vaccine production requires approval by the NRA.

An alternative to the conventional approach to reassortant development is the use of an RG methodology to produce a reassortant vaccine virus (*24*). This process usually incorporates into plasmids the six RNA segments encoding the internal proteins of a backbone donor virus and the two segments encoding the HA and NA from the WHO-recommended vaccine virus. The plasmids are subsequently transfected into cells, with or without additional helper plasmids, in order to generate the CVVs to be used for vaccine manufacturing. RG technology allows for the direct manipulation of the influenza gene segments and can be faster than the use of conventional reassortment. Moreover, if an HPAI virus is used in the RG process, the HA gene can be modified to remove the specific amino acid motif at the HA cleavage site that is known to convey high pathogenicity in poultry (*25*). The reassortant can thus be specifically designed to serve as a CVV without the capacity to cause high pathogenicity in birds. The RG system has been reported to produce a CVV within 9–12 days (*26*) but further analysis of the product takes additional time. The distribution and receipt of the WHO-recommended vaccine virus as a source of RNA for constructing RG HA and NA plasmids adds extra time to the reassortment process. These delays can be minimized if the reassorting laboratories use site-directed mutagenesis of existing plasmids containing the HA and NA genes of a related virus, or by the use of synthetic DNA (*27, 28*).

4.1.2 Backbone donor viruses

Reassortant CVVs containing donor genes – with the exception of segments 4 and 6 (HA and NA) – from backbone donor viruses (PR8, A/Ann Arbor/6/60 or

A/Leningrad/134/17/57) have been widely used to produce seasonal influenza vaccines and pandemic A(H1N1)pdm09 vaccines. A substantial body of data indicates that reassortant viruses composed of RNA segments coding for HA and NA derived from a pandemic virus or IVPP and the RNA segments coding for the internal proteins from PR8, A/Ann Arbor/6/60 or A/Leningrad/134/17/57 will have only a low probability of causing harm to human health (*10, 24*).

PR8 is a common backbone donor virus for generating reassortant vaccine viruses as it replicates to high titre in embryonated hens' eggs. Originally used in the late 1960s to produce "high-growth reassortants", the use of such reassortants as vaccine viruses increases vaccine yield many fold (*29–31*). Moreover, PR8 has undergone extensive passaging in mice, ferrets and embryonated hens' eggs. This has resulted in the complete attenuation of the virus, rendering it incapable of replicating in humans (*32, 33*). Improved backbone donor viruses are being developed in order to enhance yields for CVVs used to manufacture inactivated influenza virus vaccines. These new donor viruses may be derivations of PR8 viruses but they may also have genes from viruses other than PR8, be synthetically generated and/or be optimized for specific HA and NA subtypes (*26*). Demonstration of the adequate attenuation of CVVs using new/improved backbone donor viruses will be needed before approval for use (see section 5).

Some countries have licensed seasonal LAIVs that use reassortants with a 6:2 gene constellation based on donor viruses such as A/Ann Arbor/6/60 and A/Leningrad/134/17/57. Clinical studies of some 30 different vaccine viruses over a period of more than 40 years have demonstrated that both A/Ann Arbor/6/60-based and A/Leningrad/134/17/57-based reassortant vaccine viruses are attenuated for humans (*34, 35*). These donor viruses might also be used for developing pandemic influenza vaccines and an adequate level of attenuation has been shown for modified reassortant viruses of various subtypes (*36*). For each CVV derived from a new pandemic virus or IVPP, the level of attenuation should be verified by testing, as described below in section 5.1. A(H5N1)-specific LAIVs made from A/Ann Arbor/6/60 reassortants have been licensed for pandemic preparedness purposes in several countries.

4.1.3 Gene segments from wild-type viruses (WHO-recommended vaccine viruses)

The gene constellation of reassortant CVVs derived by traditional co-cultivation methods must be determined. Reassortants with 6:2 or 5:3 gene constellations containing the HA and NA genes of the wild-type strain are the most common – however, reassortants containing other gene combinations may also be considered. NRAs will provide guidance and give approval to acceptable gene constellations for use in influenza vaccines. It is also possible that a mutant (non-reassortant) wild-type virus could be selected that has improved growth characteristics.

Because of their potential association with pathogenicity, genes from the wild-type virus (especially the HA and NA genes) require particular attention.

4.1.3.1 Haemagglutinin cleavage site

Most HPAI viruses of the H5 and H7 subtypes contain sequences of basic amino acids at the cleavage sites separating their HA1 and HA2 domains. Elimination of these HA polybasic cleavage sites is associated with reduced virulence in mammalian and avian models and with a low IVPI. However, some wild-type LPAI viruses (for example, A(H7N9) viruses) have caused serious human disease despite causing few signs of illness in poultry (*37*).

For reassortants derived from HPAI H5 and H7 viruses by RG, the HA should be modified so that the amino acids inserted at the HA cleavage site are reduced to a single basic amino acid; additional nucleotide substitutions can be introduced in the vicinity of the cleavage site in order to increase the genetic stability of the created monobasic motif during large-scale vaccine manufacture. Cleavage site modifications have consistently reduced pathogenicity for avian embryos and poultry (*38*). However, modifying the cleavage site does not guarantee low pathogenicity in humans and other mammalian species because of the presence of other virulence factors (*39, 40*).

4.1.3.2 Receptor specificity

Preferential binding of the HA to α2,6-linked terminal sialic acid residues is associated with transmissibility of influenza viruses in humans (*41, 42*). However, viruses that preferentially bind to α2,3-linked terminal sialic acid residues (for example, A(H7N9) and A(H5N1) viruses) do not transmit well between humans but may on occasion infect humans and cause serious illness (*43*). While receptor specificity must be considered as a factor in reducing the risk of virus transmissibility and of causing harm to human health, modifying it is insufficient for virus attenuation.

The hazards associated with reassortants depend in part on HA receptor specificity. If a reassortant has a preference for avian cell receptors (that is, α2,3-linked terminal sialic acid), the hazard to humans is considered to be lower. However, if a reassortant has a preference for mammalian cell receptors (α2,6-linkages; for example, the 1957 A(H2N2) pandemic virus) or possesses both avian and mammalian receptor specificities, there is a greater risk of transmissibility and human infection. For A/goose/Guangdong/1/96-lineage H5 reassortants, it is anticipated that the HA will retain a preference for α2,3-linked terminal sialic acid residues, and so their transmissibility between humans should be reduced. However, some HPAI A(H5N1) viruses (for example, from Egypt) have been reported to exhibit increased binding to α2,6 linkages while maintaining a preference for α2,3-linked terminal sialic acid residues (*44, 45*).

WHO Technical Report Series, No. 1016, 2019

It is anticipated that A(H5N1) reassortant viruses derived by RG according to WHO guidance (*46*) would be attenuated for humans compared to wild-type H5 viruses. Nevertheless, the human lower respiratory tract contains α2,3-linked sialic acid receptors and thus exposure to high doses of A(H5N1) viruses represents a risk of infection. Moreover, humans are immunologically naive to H5 and many other avian subtypes, and this too is an important risk factor.

It should be noted that influenza virus pathogenicity does not depend solely on HA but is a polygenic trait. The 1997 A(H5N1) virus had unusual PB2 and NS1 genes that influenced pathogenicity, whereas 2004 A(H5N1) viruses possessed complex combinations of changes in different gene segments that affected their pathogenicity in ferrets (*47, 48*). Compared to HA, the NA protein of influenza viruses has a less prominent role as a virulence factor. It is known that a balance of HA (receptor binding) and NA (receptor destruction and virus release) activities is required for efficient viral replication (*49, 50*). Further, specific adaptations in NA have been identified that facilitate transmission from wild aquatic birds to poultry. However, specific NA determinants for adaptation to, and virulence in, humans have so far not been found – though there is some evidence that the NA can mediate HA cleavage in A(H1N1) viruses (*51, 52*). It is of note that resistance to the viral inhibitors oseltamivir and zanamivir is caused by specific mutations in either NA or HA. While it is acknowledged that there is a long history of safety for reassortants using PR8 or LAIV backbones, safety testing should be conducted as new CVVs are being produced (see section 5, Table A3.1 below) unless virus-specific risk assessments suggest a different approach.

4.1.3.3 Secondary reassortment

It is conceivable that reassortment between a CVV containing HA and NA from an IVPP and a human wild-type seasonal influenza virus could occur during simultaneous infection of humans with both viruses. For secondary reassortants to be generated the following would need to happen:

- infection of a human (for example, vaccine production staff) with the CVV;
- simultaneous infection of the same human with a wild-type seasonal influenza virus; and
- reassortment between the CVV and the wild-type seasonal influenza virus.

Such a secondary reassortant may have properties distinct from the seasonal virus and might still be able to replicate in humans and spread from person to person. The likelihood of such secondary reassortment is considered to be low to negligible. However, laboratory and production facilities must have biosafety control measures in place to prevent the exposure of staff to live reassortant viruses. In a case of accidental exposure, it is unlikely that a CVV would replicate efficiently or transmit to human contacts. In over 40 years of vaccine manufacturing, there have been no reported cases of influenza resulting from the secondary reassortment of CVVs.

4.1.4   Wild-type HPAI CVVs

The use of wild-type HPAI CVVs has been confined to cell-culture-based production, which for inactivated vaccines uses closed systems under high containment. Stringent biosafety and biosecurity measures are required during production, analytical testing and waste disposal in order to protect staff and prevent the release of infectious virus into the environment. CVVs produced by RG and demonstrated to be attenuated, as described in section 5 below, are preferred.

4.1.5   Other wild-type CVVs

Vaccines may also be produced from other wild-type CVVs (for example, swine and LPAI viruses).

The pathogenicity of these wild-type viruses for humans cannot be predicted; some A(H7N9) viruses that are of low pathogenicity in poultry have caused severe illness in humans (53). Although the transmissibility of wild-type viruses with avian receptor specificity is likely to be low in humans, the transmissibility of wild-type viruses with mammalian receptor specificity (for example, swine viruses) is largely unknown and is likely to depend on a number of factors, including population immunity.

Appropriate measures should be in place to prevent exposure of staff to CVVs derived from wild-type viruses because of the risk of secondary reassortment with circulating influenza viruses, as described in section 4.1.3.3.

4.1.6   Susceptibility of CVVs to NA inhibitors

CVVs that are sensitive to NA inhibitors or other licensed drugs should be used for vaccine production whenever possible. If the relationship between genotype and phenotype is well known, sequence verification may be sufficient to confirm the presence of genetic motifs known to be associated with drug susceptibility. Otherwise, susceptibility should be confirmed by phenotypic testing.

5. Safety testing of candidate vaccine viruses

CVVs can be developed by WHO GISRS laboratories, laboratories associated with WHO GISRS that have been approved by an NRA, and the laboratories of vaccine manufacturers. The following tests and specifications have been developed on the basis of experience gained in evaluating CVVs derived from viruses of various subtypes. The safety testing required for different CVVs and their proposed containment levels are summarized in Table A3.1. The information summarized in this table should be considered as guidance – changes in the requirements may be determined on a case-by-case basis by WHO and/or national authorities. For CVVs developed from newly emerging IVPP, a WHO expert group will review the data obtained from safety testing and advise WHO. WHO will then provide further guidance on appropriate containment requirements through its expert networks such as WHO GISRS. Moreover, laboratories that generate CVVs will produce a summary report of all safety testing conducted on a given CVV. This documentation may be of assistance for importation/transportation purposes and is available on request from those laboratories.

The requirement to conduct or complete some or all of these tests prior to the distribution of a CVV may be relaxed on the basis of additional risk assessments. Such assessments should take into account evolving virological, epidemiological and clinical data, and national and international regulatory requirements for the shipment and receipt of infectious substances.

Animal tests with CVVs and IVPP should be conducted in animal containment facilities in accordance with the proposed containment levels shown in Table A3.1. For untested CVVs, the containment level to be used is the one shown for the respective wild-type virus. In specific cases – such as CVVs derived from synthetic DNA encoding modified HA genes (see footnote "c" in Table A3.1) from H5 and H7 HPAI viruses – the containment level may be lowered based on a virus-specific risk assessment. An appropriate occupational health policy should be in place.

5.1 Tests to evaluate pathogenicity of candidate vaccine viruses

The recommended tests for evaluating the pathogenicity of CVVs depend on the parental wild-type viruses (that is, WHO-recommended vaccine viruses) from which they are derived (Table A3.1). The nature of the parental viruses and the risks of the procedures involved will also determine the required containment level. The tests required to evaluate CVVs are described in the following sections. Some CVVs may not require complete safety testing if they are genetically similar to a CVV that has already been tested – that is, they have HAs and NAs derived from the same (or a genetically closely related) wild-type virus and are on the same (or a genetically closely related) backbone and have the same internal gene constellation. For these CVVs, it may be sufficient to confirm sequence and genetic stability as determined by a WHO expert group and/or by competent national authorities.

5.1.1   Attenuation in ferrets

Ferrets have been used extensively as a good indicator of influenza virus virulence in humans (*54*). Typically, seasonal influenza viruses cause mild-to-no clinical signs in ferrets, and virus replication is usually limited to the respiratory tract. PR8 viruses have also been assessed in ferrets and have been found to cause few or no clinical signs, with virus replication limited to the upper respiratory tract (*39*). Conversely, some wild-type HPAI viruses can cause severe and sometimes fatal infections in ferrets (*48, 55*). Thus, in the absence of human data, the ferret is generally considered to be the best model for predicting pathogenicity and/or attenuation in humans. The mouse is not considered an appropriate model for the safety testing of influenza CVVs.

CVVs should be shown to be attenuated in ferrets in accordance with Table A3.1, except when virus-specific risk assessments suggest a different approach (for example, waiving the ferret test where Table A3.1 requires it). These tests should be conducted in well-characterized and standardized ferret models (for example, by using common reference viruses, when available, from WHO collaborating centres and/or essential regulatory laboratories for influenza). Detailed test procedures are described in Appendix 1 of these WHO Guidelines. One or more laboratories may have ferret pathogenicity data on parental wild-type viruses (that is, WHO-recommended vaccine viruses) that could be used by all testing laboratories as a further benchmark for comparison. Limiting the testing requirements for the wild-type viruses will help counteract the time delays associated with the export and import of IVPP and/or pandemic viruses. Assessing the transmissibility of CVVs between ferrets is not required because of the difficulties of standardizing this assay across laboratories (*56, 57*).

5.1.2   Pathogenicity in chickens

For CVVs derived from HPAI H5 or H7 parental viruses, determination of the chicken IVPI is recommended and may also be required by national authorities. The procedure should follow that described in OIE guidance (*58*). Any virus with an index greater than 1.2, or that causes at least 75% mortality in inoculated chickens, is considered to be an HPAI virus (*58*).

5.1.3   The ability of virus to plaque in the presence or absence of added trypsin

HPAI viruses replicate in mammalian cell culture in the absence of added trypsin – whereas LPAI viruses generally do not. This test is recommended for all CVVs derived from HPAI H5 or H7 parental viruses. It is recommended that the test be established and characterized using known positive and negative control viruses (*59*).

WHO Technical Report Series, No. 1016, 2019

<h3>5.1.4   Gene sequencing</h3>

Gene sequencing is required for confirming virus identity and/or verifying the presence of attenuating and other phenotypic markers (for example, markers of cold adaptation and temperature sensitivity in the case of LAIV CVVs). HA and NA genes should be fully sequenced, with the extent of backbone gene segment sequencing dependent on the nature of the backbone donor viruses (for example, LAIV CVVs may require full sequencing to confirm the presence of attenuating mutations).

<h3>5.1.5   Genetic stability</h3>

The genetic stability of CVVs is generally assessed after 6–10 passages in relevant substrates (that is, embryonated hens' eggs or cultured cells). Subsequent sequence analysis can verify the retention (stability) of the markers of relevant phenotypic traits related to pathogenicity, where such markers are known. These tests should be conducted on all CVVs (including wild-type CVVs) prepared from pandemic viruses and IVPP. It may be possible to ship viruses to manufacturers before genetic stability has been fully established by the reassorting laboratories.

Table A3.1

Required safety testing of CVVs and proposed containment levels for vaccine production

Category of CVV	Tests needed on CVVs[a]	Proposed containment level for vaccine production[b]
Modified reassortant viruses based on H5 and H7 HPAI viruses[c]	Ferret (5.1.1); chicken (5.1.2);[d] plaquing (5.1.3); sequence (5.1.4); genetic stability (5.1.5)[e]	BSL2 enhanced (6.5.1)
Reassortant viruses derived from H5 and H7 LPAI viruses	Ferret (5.1.1); sequence (5.1.4); genetic stability (5.1.5)[e]	BSL2 enhanced (6.5.1)
Reassortant viruses derived from non-H5 or non-H7 viruses	Ferret (5.1.1); sequence (5.1.4); genetic stability (5.1.5)[e]	BSL2 enhanced (6.5.1)
Wild-type H5, H7 HPAI viruses	Sequence (5.1.4); genetic stability (5.1.5);[e] also see footnote f	BSL3 enhanced (6.4)
Wild-type H5, H7 LPAI viruses	Ferret (5.1.1); sequence (5.1.4); genetic stability (5.1.5);[e] also see footnote g	BSL2 enhanced (6.5.1)[g]

Table A3.1 *continued*

Category of CVV	Tests needed on CVVs[a]	Proposed containment level for vaccine production[b]
Wild-type non-H5 or non-H7 viruses	Ferret (5.1.1); sequence (5.1.4); genetic stability (5.1.5);[e] also see footnote g	BSL2 enhanced (6.5.1)[g]

[a] Tests to be performed by a WHO GISRS or other approved laboratory.

[b] The proposed containment levels may be changed (to higher or lower containment) based on a specific risk assessment.

[c] This category refers to viruses derived by RG technology such that the additional amino acids at the HA cleavage site are removed.

[d] The requirement for performance of the chicken pathogenicity test (IVPI) is dependent on national regulatory requirements which are currently under review in some countries and may change.

[e] Genetic stability testing should be performed. However, it should not delay the distribution and use of the CVV by manufacturers and can be performed subsequently.

[f] Testing in ferrets and chicken (IVPI) is not required because the highly pathogenic phenotype is already known and the highest containment level is required to work with these viruses.

[g] If a virus-specific hazard assessment identifies that additional control measures are appropriate, the containment level may be increased. The requirements for this level may be specific to a particular facility and should be assessed on a case-by-case basis by the relevant competent national authority.

6. Risk assessment and management

6.1   Nature of the work

Influenza vaccine production in embryonated hens' eggs or cell culture requires the propagation of live virus. In most cases, the generation of CVVs will result in viruses that are expected to be attenuated in humans (*10, 24*). Several steps in the manufacturing process have the potential to generate aerosols containing live virus. The virus concentration in aerosols will depend on the specific production step and will be highest during the harvesting of infectious allantoic fluid and much lower during seed virus preparation and egg inoculation (which involve either small amounts of liquid containing virus or very dilute virus suspensions). Appropriate biosafety measures (for example, the use of laminar air flows, biological safety cabinets with HEPA filtration, cleaning and decontamination of equipment, waste management and spill kits) must be in place to prevent accidental exposure in the work environment and the release of virus into the general environment.

6.2   Health protection

6.2.1   Likelihood of harm to human health

Wild-type influenza viruses are able to infect humans and cause serious illness – however, many of the viruses used for producing vaccines are CVVs in an attenuating donor backbone (for example, A/PR/8/34, A/Ann Arbor/6/60 or A/Leningrad/134/17/57) and so the resulting CVV will have a low probability of causing harm to human health.

Vaccine manufacture requires adherence to both GMP and appropriate biosafety requirements for biological products, as well as to related national regulations, technical standards and guidelines. GMP protects the product from the operator, and protects the operator and the environment from the infectious agent, thus reducing the risk of any hazard associated with production. Reassortants derived from PR8 backbone donor viruses have been used routinely for producing inactivated influenza vaccines for over 40 years. This work usually requires thousands of litres of infectious egg allantoic fluid, which can create substantial aerosols of reassortant virus within manufacturing plants. Although manufacturing staff may be susceptible to infection with these virus aerosols, there have been no documented or anecdotal cases of work-related human illness resulting from occupational exposure to the reassortant viruses described above. Similarly, reassortants derived from the A/Ann Arbor/6/60 and A/Leningrad/134/17/57 viruses have been used for the production of LAIV for many years with no reported cases of work-related human illness related to these viruses. While no study has yet been undertaken to detect asymptomatic infections caused by either PR8-derived or live attenuated viruses, the attenuation status of these CVVs continues to be supported by their excellent safety record.

The use of pandemic CVVs that express avian influenza genes may lead to potential consequences for agricultural systems. For example, if influenza A H5 or H7 viruses or any influenza A virus with an IVPI greater than 1.2 are introduced into poultry (60) then OIE must be notified of the presence of infection, and this could lead to the implementation of biosecurity measures aimed at preventing the spread of disease (58, 60). Moreover, infection of birds other than poultry (including wild birds) with influenza A viruses of high pathogenicity must also be reported to OIE.

6.2.2   Vaccine production in eggs

Influenza vaccine has been produced in embryonated hens' eggs since the early 1940s. Much experience has been gained since then, with some facilities capable of handling large numbers of eggs on a daily basis with the aid of mechanized egg-handling, inoculation and harvesting machines.

Hazards may occur during production stages and/or laboratory quality control activities prior to virus inactivation. During egg inoculation only small amounts of liquid containing virus or very dilute virus suspensions are used. When the eggs are opened to harvest the allantoic fluid, the open nature of this operation may result in hazardous exposure to aerosols and spills. Following this step, the allantoic fluid is handled in closed vessels and so the hazards arising from live virus during subsequent processing and virus inactivation (if used) are less than during virus harvest. The collection and disposal of egg waste is potentially a significant environmental hazard. Ensuring the safe disposal of the waste from egg-grown vaccines, both within the plant and outside, is therefore critical and procedures should comply with the guidance and/or requirements of competent national authorities.

6.2.3 Vaccine production in cell culture

For pandemic influenza vaccines produced in cell cultures, the biosafety risks associated with manufacturing will depend primarily on the nature of the cell culture system. Closed systems such as bioreactors usually present little or no opportunity for exposure to live virus during normal operation – however, additional safety measures must be taken during procedures for adding samples to the bioreactor or removing them from it. Virus production in roller bottles and cell culture flasks may allow for exposure to live virus through aerosols, spills and other means. Additional risks can be associated with the inactivation and disposal of the large quantities of contaminated liquid and solid waste (including cellular debris) generated by this method.

During passage in mammalian cells, it is possible that genetic mutations may be selected for in pandemic and IVPP CVVs that render them more adapted to humans. These changes are most likely to occur within or close to the receptor-binding domain of the HA glycoprotein. Sequence analysis may detect such changes, but whether these changes affect the ability of a mutant virus to cause infection in humans is not well established. In one study, an attempt to de-attenuate a PR8 virus by multiple passage in organ cultures of human tissue failed (*32*). Another study showed that human viruses with α2,6 receptor specificity were likely to mutate to α2,3 receptor specificity upon passage in Madin-Darby Canine Kidney (MDCK) cells thus making them less likely to be infectious for humans (*61*). Overall, the hazards arising from the inherent properties of a reassortant or wild-type virus are likely to be greater than the probability of the virus adapting to a more human-like phenotype in cell culture.

6.2.4 Hazards from the vaccine

Inactivated pandemic influenza vaccines present no biosafety risks beyond the manufacturing process, provided that the results of the inactivation steps show complete virus inactivation, rendering the virus incapable of replication.

In an interpandemic or pandemic alert phase, pilot-scale live attenuated pandemic influenza vaccines may be developed for clinical evaluation. The biosafety risks associated with virus shedding or other unintentional release of virus into the environment following vaccination should be carefully assessed. Based on this risk assessment, subjects participating in clinical trials in the

WHO Technical Report Series, No. 1016, 2019

interpandemic or pandemic alert phases should be kept in clinical isolation. If this is not done then indirect hazards for humans could arise.

While it is very unlikely that an LAIV will be harmful to humans, an indirect potential hazard may exist through secondary reassortment with a human or animal influenza virus, as discussed in section 4.1.3.3.

Evidence to date indicates that the probability of generating secondary reassortants is very low (62). Moreover, containment procedures have significantly improved over the last 40 years and production staff can be vaccinated to reduce the chances of acquiring an infection with a circulating wild-type seasonal influenza virus, thus minimizing the risk of secondary reassortment. In addition, appropriate personal protective equipment (PPE) can also be provided.

6.3 Environmental protection

6.3.1 Environmental considerations

Influenza A viruses are enzootic or epizootic in some farm animals (poultry, pigs and horses) and in some populations of wild birds – particularly birds of the families Anseriformes (ducks, geese and swans) and Charadriiformes (shorebirds) (63).

Several avian influenza A viruses (especially H5 and H7 subtypes) can be highly pathogenic in poultry. In addition, sporadic infections by influenza A viruses have been reported in other species, including farmed mink, wild whales, seals, captive populations of wild cats (tigers and leopards) (64) and domestic cats (65) and dogs (66). In big cats, infection has been reported following the consumption of dead chickens infected with A(H5N1) viruses.

It is expected that many IVPP will have avian receptor specificity and thus birds would theoretically be most susceptible. Many studies indicate that viruses with PR8 backbones are attenuated in chickens. For example, a reassortant containing an HA with a single basic amino acid at the cleavage site, an NA from the 1997 Hong Kong A(H5N1) virus and the genes coding for the internal protein genes of a PR8 virus was barely able to replicate in chickens and was not lethal (67). Similarly, a 6:2 PR8 reassortant that contained a 2003 Hong Kong A(H5N1) HA did not replicate or cause signs of disease in chickens (39). The removal of the multiple basic amino acids at the HA cleavage site in these H5/PR8 reassortants probably played a major role in reducing the risk for chickens.

It is likely that the temperature-sensitive phenotype of cold-adapted vaccine viruses would limit replication of these viruses in avian species due to the higher body temperature of birds. Pigs, however, have both $\alpha 2,3$- and $\alpha 2,6$-linked sialic acid receptors in abundance (68) and, in the absence of direct evidence to the contrary, must be considered susceptible to most influenza A viruses, including LAIV and PR8 reassortants.

6.4 Assignment of containment level

Definition of the required containment conditions must be based on an activity-based risk assessment, taking into account the scale of manipulations, the titres of live virus and whether an activity involves virus amplification. Biosafety control measures must be reconciled with rules and regulations governing the manufacture and testing of medicinal products under GMP (*69*). It should be noted that biosafety control measures apply to manipulations involving live virus – such measures no longer apply once a virus has been inactivated by a validated process.

The generation of reassortant CVVs from HPAI viruses typically takes place in BSL3 facilities, as advised by WHO (*46*), with additional enhancements (BSL3 enhanced). The use of additional physical and/or operational precautions, above those described for BSL3 (*11*), should be based on a local risk assessment in consultation with the competent national authority and/or regulatory authority. The specific enhancements will vary from facility to facility and will depend on the design of the facility and operational procedures employed. Such enhancements may include the use of dedicated laboratory clothing, availability of shower facilities, final HEPA filtration of laboratory exhaust air, laboratory effluent decontamination and a quarantine plan.

Special consideration should be given to the hazards associated with the cell-culture production and quality control of vaccines made from HPAI wild-type CVVs. In view of the open nature of large-scale egg-based vaccine production, it is not feasible to operate in BSL3 enhanced conditions. Therefore, egg-based vaccine production from HPAI wild-type viruses is not recommended.

Because of the hazards associated with egg- and cell-culture vaccine production and quality control involving the use of conventional or RG-derived reassortant CVVs that are known to be attenuated (see section 5.1), the production facility should have a BSL2 enhanced containment level, as specified in section 6.5.1. Under defined circumstances, CVVs for which safety testing has not yet been completed may be used in production facilities that comply with containment level BSL2 enhanced with additional controls, as specified in section 6.5.2, with the approval of the NRA. The parts of the facility where such work (both production and quality control) is carried out should meet national and OIE requirements for containment. These requirements include biosafety and biosecurity requirements and environmental controls that limit the introduction into, and spread within, animal populations (*58*). The requirements to be met should be agreed upon with WHO and competent national and regional authorities (*19, 70*). This guidance applies to both pilot-scale and large-scale production during the interpandemic and pandemic alert phases (*19*). Any subsequent relaxation of the containment level to the standard used for seasonal vaccine production must be authorized by the competent national authorities on a case-by-case basis after evaluating the risks.

6.5 Environmental control measures

Containment measures to prevent the release of live virus into the environment should be established on the basis of a risk assessment specific to the virus, the production system and relevant biosafety guidelines – either those of NRAs or of WHO.

Local biosafety and biosecurity regulations provide guidance on the disposal of potentially infectious waste. In particular, contaminated waste from production facilities may reach very high virus titres. All decontamination methods should be validated at regular intervals as required by the competent national authority. If possible, decontamination of waste should take place on site. Where this is not possible, it is the responsibility of the manufacturer to contain material safely during transport prior to off-site decontamination. Guidance on regulations for the transport of infectious substances is available from WHO (*18*) and from competent national authorities. In all cases, procedures must be validated to ensure that they function at the scale of manufacturing. Stringent measures to control rodents, other mammals and birds must also be in place.

Each manufacturer should also assess the risk of exposing birds, horses, pigs or other susceptible animals if they are likely to be in the vicinity of the manufacturing plant. Following potential occupational exposure to live virus, staff or other personnel should avoid visiting pig, horse or bird facilities (for example, farms, equestrian events and bird sanctuaries) for at least 14 days following exposure. If conjunctivitis or respiratory signs and symptoms suggest that influenza might develop during this 14-day period, the quarantine period should be extended to 14 days (twice the expected time for virus shedding) after the signs and symptoms have resolved (*71*).

6.5.1 Specifications for BSL2 enhanced production facilities

In addition to the principles for BSL2 facilities specified in the WHO *Laboratory biosafety manual* (*11*), the specifications for BSL2 enhanced facilities include those described below.

6.5.1.1 Facility

The facility should be designed and operated in such a way as to protect the vaccine, the staff producing and testing the vaccine, the environment and the population at large. Different solutions may be needed according to the risks inherent in the operation(s) conducted in the area. Specialized engineering solutions will be required that may include the following:

- Use of relative negative pressure biosafety cabinets;
- HEPA filtration of air prior to its exhaust into public areas or the environment;

- Room pressure cascades designed to contain live virus safely while also protecting the product. A net negative pressure between the atmosphere and areas where live virus is handled can be separated by an area (barrier) of positive pressure higher than the pressure both in the atmosphere and in areas where live virus is handled. Alternatively, a negative-pressure barrier can be built where live virus is trapped and then removed by HEPA filtration before it can escape into the atmosphere.

In addition, the following decontamination procedures should take place:

- decontamination of all waste from BSL2 enhanced (pandemic influenza vaccine) areas; and

- decontamination of all potentially contaminated areas at the end of a production campaign through cleaning and validated decontamination measures (for example, fumigation).

6.5.1.2 Personal protection

A range of personal protection measures should be in place, including the following:

- Full-body protective laboratory clothing (for example, Tyvek® disposable overalls) should be available.

- If activities cannot be contained by primary containment and open activities are being conducted, the use of respiratory protective equipment which can be checked for close facial fit – such as FFP2 (for example, N95) or FFP3 (*72*) respirators – is required. Appropriate minimum specifications for the filtering/absorbing capacity of such equipment should be met and masks, if used, must be fitted properly and the correctness of fit tested.

- All personnel, including support staff and others who may enter the production or quality control areas where CVVs, pandemic viruses and IVPP are handled, should sign a written document in which they agree not to have any contact with susceptible animals (for example, ferrets or farm animals, especially birds, horses and pigs) for 14 days after leaving the facility where vaccine has been produced. If conjunctivitis or respiratory signs and symptoms suggest that influenza might develop during this 14-day period, the quarantine period should be extended to 14 days (twice the expected time for virus shedding) after the signs and symptoms have resolved (*71*). Currently the risks involved in contact with household dogs and cats are not considered to be significant, but the scientific evidence on this risk is sparse.

- It is strongly recommended that staff should be vaccinated with seasonal influenza vaccines.

- If vaccines targeting the virus in production are available and marketing authorization has been received, vaccination with these vaccines is recommended for staff before large-scale vaccine production commences.

- A medical surveillance programme for staff should be established prior to manufacturing activities. Antiviral medicines should always be available in case of accidental exposure. Where these medicines are available only on prescription, access to prescribing doctors/ hospitals and to stocks of medication should be ensured.

6.5.1.3   Monitoring of decontamination

Cleaning and decontamination methods must be validated and reviewed periodically as part of a master plan to demonstrate that the protocols, reagents and equipment used are effective in inactivating pandemic influenza virus on all surfaces, garments of personnel, waste materials and storage containers. Once decontamination protocols for influenza virus have been fully described and validated, there is no need to conduct a separate validation study for each new influenza virus. Validation studies using influenza viruses may be supplemented by studies with biological (for example, bacterial) markers selected to be more difficult to inactivate than influenza virus.

6.5.2   Specifications for BSL2 enhanced production facilities with additional controls

It is assumed that ferret pathogenicity testing will be conducted on all CVVs of unknown pathogenicity, even given the assumptions outlined above (see section 5.1) regarding the low probability that a PR8 reassortant virus or LAIV is pathogenic for humans. This assumption is based on current experience in relation to reassortants of HA subtypes other than H1 and H3 (that is, H5, H7 and H9). A facility must meet the requirements for protecting personnel who handle potentially dangerous microorganisms. The WHO *Laboratory biosafety manual* (*11*) includes a risk survey that can be undertaken prior to rating a laboratory space as BSL1, BSL2 or BSL3. Similar requirements can be found in Directive 2000/54/EC of the European Parliament and of the Council (70) on the protection of workers from risks related to exposure to biological agents at work, and the United States Department of Health and Human Services *Biosafety in microbiological and biomedical laboratories* (5th edition) (*72*).

Large-scale vaccine manufacturing using a CVV before its safety testing is complete can be considered if justified by evolving virological, epidemiological and clinical data, and if it meets national and international regulatory requirements regarding the shipment, receipt and handling of infectious substances.

A facility that meets the criteria detailed below in section 6.5.2.1 and that has the noted operator protections in place could be considered suitable for manufacturing vaccine at large scale using a CVV prepared by RG or a conventional reassortant methodology before safety testing is complete, with the approval of the NRA.

6.5.2.1 Facility

The facility should be designed and operated in such a way as to protect the vaccine, the staff producing and testing the vaccine, the environment and the population at large. This will require specialized engineering solutions that may include the following:

- Appropriate signage and labelling must be in place regarding the activities being carried out when a virus is in use while the safety testing is being completed.

- The facility must be designed and constructed as a contained GMP space. The surfaces and finishes must comply with GMP requirements (69) that ensure they can be sealed and easily cleaned and decontaminated.

- The air cascades within the facility should be such that any live virus can be contained within the work zones in which it is being used. All work with infectious virus must be conducted within these contained zones.

- Access to the contained areas must be via double-door entry airlocks. The airlocks should operate at a pressure that is either lower or higher than that on either side. In this way the airlocks become either a "sink" or a pressure barrier, containing the flow of air within the facility. In cases where the airlocks provide a low-pressure sink, the entry and exit doors should be interlocked or fitted with a suitable delay or alarm system to prevent both being opened at the same time. It is also acceptable if the airlocks are part of a series of increasing negative pressure. The air pressure cascade within the negative-pressure contained zone should comply with GMP requirements (that is, higher pressures in cleanest zones) for clean rooms.

- All supply and exhaust air must be passed through HEPA filtration while maintaining all required containment and GMP conditions.

WHO Technical Report Series, No. 1016, 2019

Air-handling systems within the facility must be rigorously assessed to ensure that they protect against potential failure. Fail-safe systems must be installed wherever necessary. The facility should be constantly monitored to ensure that appropriate room pressure differentials are maintained.

- All reusable equipment should be cleaned in place, decontaminated by means of autoclaving, or otherwise cleaned and decontaminated by validated, dedicated systems prior to reuse.

- Areas of potential liquid spill, including waste-treatment plants and processes, should be assessed and bunded to ensure that any spill is contained. Procedures must be in place to ensure that spills are contained, areas are cleaned and contaminated materials are properly disposed of in order not to compromise the integrity of the facility.

- The entry of materials into contained zones should be via separately HEPA-filtered, interlocked, double-ended "pass-through cabinets" or double-ended autoclaves.

- All facility waste, including egg waste, should be discarded via validated on-site waste-effluent systems or following decontamination by autoclaving. Any items which pass from the external environment to the manufacturing process and are later returned to the external environment (for example, egg trays) must receive special attention. Dedicated procedures for the washing and decontamination of equipment must be in place and fully validated.

6.5.2.2 Personal protection

- All clothing worn outside the facility should be replaced by manufacturing-facility garments on entry into the facility.

- Gowning in areas in which live virus is handled should always include full suit, overshoes, eye protection and double gloves.

- Suitable PPE (full hood powered air-purifying respirators based on the risk assessment) should be provided for all personnel working in containment areas within the manufacturing facility. The hoods should be worn at all times when the facility is in operation under these enhanced biosafety requirements.

- All facility clothing is to be removed on exit, with soiled clothing removed from the facility via a decontamination autoclave or similar method. The surfaces of respirator hoods should be decontaminated.

- Specific procedures should be developed and implemented for the operation of the facility under enhanced biosecurity conditions.

- It is strongly recommended that staff should be vaccinated with a seasonal influenza vaccine. In the case of pandemic viruses and IVPP, and before large-scale vaccine production is attempted, pilot lots of vaccine may already have been produced. If they are available and if marketing authorization has been received, vaccination of staff against the virus being produced is recommended before large-scale production begins.

- Procedures should be in place to provide antiviral treatment whenever warranted (for example, following accidental exposure).

- On-site occupational health and safety and medical support should be maximized by providing medical consultation and training in recognizing influenza-like symptoms, along with out-of-hours referral to medical facilities with quarantine capabilities.

- It is recommended that staff should take showers on exiting the facility. Showers are mandatory for staff who may have been accidently exposed to vaccine virus.

- All personnel, including support staff and others who may enter the production or quality control areas where CVVs, pandemic viruses and IVPP are handled, should sign a written document in which they agree not to have any contact with susceptible animals (for example, ferrets or farm animals, especially birds, horses and pigs) for 14 days after leaving the facility where vaccine has been produced. If conjunctivitis or respiratory signs and symptoms suggest that influenza might develop during this 14-day period, the quarantine period should be extended to 14 days (twice the expected time for virus shedding) after the signs and symptoms have resolved (*71*). Currently the risks involved in contact with household dogs and cats are not considered to be significant, but the scientific evidence on this risk is sparse.

6.6 Biosafety management and implementation within a vaccine production facility

6.6.1 Management structure

The implementation of these WHO Guidelines requires that the institution employs a biosafety officer who is knowledgeable about large-scale virus production and containment but whose reporting responsibilities are independent of the production unit. The biosafety officer is responsible for overseeing the implementation of biosafety practices, policies and emergency procedures within the company or organization and should report directly to the highest management level. A biosafety officer is needed in addition to a qualified person who, in some countries, has overall responsibility for a medicinal product.

A biosafety committee that includes representatives of the vaccine production and quality control units should be responsible for reviewing the biosafety status of the company and for coordinating preventive and corrective measures. The institutional biosafety officer must be a member of the committee. The committee chairperson should be independent of both the production and quality control units. The biosafety committee should report to the executive management of the manufacturing company to ensure that adequate priority is given to the implementation of the required biosafety measures, and that the necessary resources are made available.

6.6.2   Medical surveillance

Manufacturers of vaccines to protect against human pandemic influenza viruses and IVPP should provide training to their occupational health professionals in recognizing the clinical signs and symptoms of influenza. Company physicians, nurses and vaccine manufacturing supervisors and staff must make decisions on the health of personnel who are associated with the manufacturing and testing of these vaccines. Local medical practitioners caring for personnel from the manufacturing site should receive special training in the diagnosis and management of pandemic influenza infection and should have access to rapid influenza diagnostic kits and to a laboratory that performs molecular diagnosis of influenza (for example, using real-time polymerase chain reaction). Any manufacturer starting large-scale production should have documented procedures – including diagnostic procedures and prescribed treatment protocols – for dealing with influenza-like illness affecting the staff and their family members. Manufacturers should ensure that staff understand their obligation to seek medical attention for any influenza-like illness and to report it to the occupational health department or equivalent. Manufacturers should ensure that antiviral treatment is available if warranted (for example, in the case of accidental exposure) and should have defined arrangements for advising staff with any influenza-like illness.

6.6.3   Implementation

A comprehensive risk analysis should be conducted to define possible sources of contamination of personnel or the environment that may arise from the production or testing of live influenza virus. The analysis should take into account the concentration, volume and stability of the virus at the site, the potential for inhalation or injection that could result from accidents, and the potential consequences of a major or minor system failure. The procedural and technical measures necessary to reduce the risk to workers and to the environment should be considered as part of this analysis, and the results should be documented.

A comprehensive biosafety manual or equivalent document must be published and implemented. The manual should fully describe the biosafety aspects of the production process and quality control activities. It should define such items as emergency procedures, waste disposal, and the safety practices and procedures that were identified in the risk analysis. The manual must be made available to all staff working in the production and quality control units, and at least one copy must be present in the containment area(s). The manual should be reviewed at least every 2 years.

Comprehensive guidelines outlining the response to biosafety emergencies, spills and accidents should be prepared and should be made available to key personnel both for information and for coordination with emergency response units. Rehearsals of emergency response procedures are helpful. The guidelines should be reviewed and updated at a defined frequency (for example, annually).

Implementation of the appropriate biosafety level in the production and testing facilities should be verified through an independent assessment. National requirements concerning verification mechanisms should be in place and must be followed.

Authors and acknowledgements

The first draft of these WHO Guidelines was prepared by Dr G. Grohmann, Environmental Pathogens, Australia and Dr T.Q. Zhou, World Health Organization, Switzerland, with critical input from Dr O.G. Engelhardt, National Institute for Biological Standards and Control, the United Kingdom; Dr J.M. Katz, Centers for Disease Control and Prevention, the USA; Dr R. Webby, St. Jude Children's Research Hospital, the USA; and Dr J. Weir, United States Food and Drug Administration, the USA, based upon inputs received during a WHO working group meeting on revision of WHO Technical Report Series 941, Annex 5: WHO biosafety risk assessment and guidelines for the production and quality control of human influenza pandemic vaccines, held in Geneva, Switzerland, 9–10 May 2017 and attended by: Dr O.G. Engelhardt, National Institute for Biological Standards and Control, the United Kingdom; Dr G. Gifford, World Organisation for Animal Health, France; Dr S. Itamura, National Institute of Infectious Diseases, Japan; Dr J.M. Katz, Centers for Disease Control and Prevention, the USA; Dr C. Li, National Institutes for Food and Drug Control, China; Dr J. McCauley, Francis Crick Institute, the United Kingdom; Dr J. Mihowich, Public Health Agency of Canada, Canada; Dr R. Wagner, Paul-Ehrlich-Institut, Germany; Dr R. Webby, St. Jude Children's Research Hospital, the USA; Dr J. Weir, Unites States Food and Drug Administration, the USA; Dr G. Zimmer, Institute of Virology and Immunology, Switzerland; and Dr M. Chafai, Dr G. Grohmann, Dr I. Knezevic, Dr W. Zhang and Dr T.Q. Zhou, World

Health Organization, Switzerland; *representatives of the International Federation of Pharmaceutical Manufacturers & Associations (IFPMA)*: Dr M. Downham, AstraZeneca/MedImmune, the United Kingdom; Dr L. Gerentes, Sanofi Pasteur, France; Dr E. Neumeier, GSK Vaccines, Germany; and Dr B. Taylor, Seqirus, the United Kingdom; *representatives of the Developing Countries Vaccine Manufacturers Network (DCVMN)*: Dr P. Patel, Cadila Healthcare Limited, India; and Dr K. Poopipatpol and Dr P. Wirachwong, Government Pharmaceutical Organization, Thailand.

Acknowledgments are also due to the following experts and institutes who provided written comments in response to the posting of the first draft document on the WHO Biologicals website for the first round of public consultation between November 2017 and February 2018: Ms P. Barbosa (*provided the consolidated comments of the IFPMA*); Mr D. Laframboise, Public Health Agency of Canada, Canada; PT Bio Farma (Persero), Indonesia; Dr R. Shivji, European Medicines Agency, the United Kingdom; Dr J. Southern, Medicines Control Council, South Africa; Dr C. Thompson and Dr M. Zambon, Public Health England, the United Kingdom; Dr T.M. Tumpey, Centers for Disease Control and Prevention, the USA; comments collected by Dr R. Donis, Biomedical Advanced Research and Development Authority, the USA (including comments from Mr M. Sharkey, Aveshka, Inc., the USA and Dr R. Fisher, the USA); Dr L.R. Yeolekar, Serum Institute of India, India; the WHO Vaccines Assessment Group, WHO Prequalification Team, World Health Organization, Switzerland; and Dr K. Kojima, Biosafety Group, World Health Organization, Switzerland.

A second draft was prepared by Dr G. Grohmann, Environmental Pathogens, Australia and Dr T.Q. Zhou, World Health Organization, Switzerland, with critical input from Dr O.G. Engelhardt, National Institute for Biological Standards and Control, the United Kingdom; Dr J.M. Katz, Centers for Disease Control and Prevention, the USA; Dr R. Webby, St. Jude Children's Research Hospital, the USA; and Dr J. Weir, United States Food and Drug Administration, the USA, taking into consideration the outcomes of a WHO informal consultation on WHO biosafety risk assessment and guidelines for the production and quality control of novel human influenza candidate vaccine viruses and pandemic vaccines, held in Geneva, Switzerland, 23–24 April 2018 and attended by: Mr P. Akarapanon, Ministry of Public Health, Thailand; Dr D. Bucher, New York Medical College, the USA; Dr O.G. Engelhardt, National Institute for Biological Standards and Control, the United Kingdom; Dr G. Grohmann, Environmental Pathogens, Australia; Dr S. Gupta, National Centre for Disease Control, India; Dr S. Itamura, National Institute of Infectious Diseases, Japan; Mr D. Laframboise, Public Health Agency of Canada, Canada; Dr J. McCauley, Francis Crick Institute, the United Kingdom; Dr G. Pavade, World Organisation for Animal Health, France; Dr M. Sergeeva, Ministry of Health of Russia, Russian Federation; Dr J. Shin,

World Health Organization Regional Office for the Western Pacific, Philippines; Dr N.T.T. Thuy, Drug Registration Division, Viet Nam; Dr R. Wagner, Paul-Ehrlich-Institut, Germany; Dr D. Wang, Chinese Center for Disease Control and Prevention, China; Dr R. Webby, St. Jude Children's Research Hospital, the USA; Dr J. Weir, United States Food and Drug Administration, the USA; Dr J. Yoon, Ministry of Food and Drug Safety, Republic of Korea; Dr M. Zambon, Public Health England, the United Kingdom; and Dr K. Kojima, Dr I. Knezevic, Dr W. Zhang and Dr T.Q. Zhou, World Health Organization, Switzerland; *representatives of the IFPMA*: Dr M. Downham, AstraZeneca/MedImmune, the United Kingdom; Dr L. Gerentes, Sanofi Pasteur, France; Dr E. Neumeier, GSK Vaccines, Germany; and Dr B. Taylor, Seqirus, the United Kingdom; *representatives of the DCVMN (including WHO pandemic influenza Global Action Plan manufacturers)*: Dr L. Yeolekar, Serum Institute of India, India; Dr I.G. Setiadi, PT Bio Farma (Persero), Indonesia; Ms V. Fongaro Botosso, Instituto Butantan, Brazil; and Dr D. Huu Thai, Institute of Vaccines and Medical Biologicals, Viet Nam.

Acknowledgments are also due to the following experts who provided written comments in response to the posting of the resulting document WHO/BS/2018.2349 on the WHO Biologicals website for a second round of public consultation from July to September 2018: Dr D. Laframboise, Public Health Agency of Canada, Canada; Dr J. Southern, Advisor to the South African Health Products Regulatory Authority, South Africa; Dr A.K. Tahlan and Dr V. Kumaresan, Central Research Institute, India; and Dr P. Barbosa (*provided the consolidated comments of the IFPMA*). Changes were then made to document WHO/BS/2018.2349 by: Dr O.G. Engelhardt, National Institute for Biological Standards and Control, the United Kingdom; Dr G. Grohmann, Environmental Pathogens, Australia; Dr J.M. Katz, Centers for Disease Control and Prevention, the USA; Dr R. Webby, St. Jude Children's Research Hospital, the USA; Dr J. Weir, United States Food and Drug Administration, the USA and Dr T.Q. Zhou, World Health Organization, Switzerland.

Further changes were subsequently made to document WHO/BS/2018.2349 by the WHO Expert Committee on Biological Standardization.

References

1. WHO biosafety risk assessment and guidelines for the production and quality control of human influenza pandemic vaccines. In: WHO Expert Committee on Biological Standardization: fifty-sixth report. Geneva: World Health Organization; 2007: Annex 5 (WHO Technical Report Series, No. 941; http://www.who.int/biologicals/publications/trs/areas/vaccines/influenza/Annex%205%20human%20pandemic%20influenza.pdf, accessed 22 January 2019).

2. Update of WHO biosafety risk assessment and guidelines for the production and quality control of human influenza pandemic vaccines. Geneva: World Health Organization; 2009 (http://www.who.int/entity/biologicals/publications/trs/areas/vaccines/influenza/H1N1_vaccine_production_biosafety_SHOC.27May2009.pdf?ua=1, accessed 22 January 2019).

3. Update of WHO biosafety risk assessment and guidelines for the production and quality control of human influenza vaccines against avian influenza A(H7N9) virus. Geneva: World Health Organization; 2013 (http://www.who.int/biologicals/BIOSAFETY_RISK_ASSESSMENT_21_MAY_2013.pdf?%2520ua, accessed 22 January 2019).

4. Influenza [website]. Geneva: World Health Organization (http://www.who.int/influenza/en/, accessed 22 January 2019).

5. Global Action Plan for Influenza Vaccines (GAP) [website]. Geneva: World Health Organization (http://www.who.int/influenza_vaccines_plan/en/, accessed 22 January 2019).

6. Influenza vaccine response during the start of a pandemic. Report of a WHO informal consultation held in Geneva, Switzerland, 29 June–1 July 2015. Geneva: World Health Organization; 2016 (Document WHO/OHE/PED/GIP/2016.1; http://apps.who.int/iris/bitstream/10665/207751/1/WHO_OHE_PED_GIP_2016.1_eng.pdf?ua=1, accessed 22 January 2019).

7. Influenza vaccine response during the start of a pandemic. Report of the second WHO informal consultation held in Geneva, Switzerland, 21–22 July 2016. Geneva: World Health Organization; 2017 (Document WHO/HSE/PED/GIP/EPI/2017.1; http://apps.who.int/iris/bitstream/handle/10665/254743/WHO-HSE-PED-GIP-EPI-2017.1-eng.pdf?sequence=1, accessed 22 January 2019).

8. WHO working group meeting on revision of WHO TRS 941, Annex 5: WHO biosafety risk assessment and guidelines for the production and quality control of human influenza pandemic vaccines. Geneva, Switzerland, 9–10 May 2017. Geneva: World Health Organization; 2017 (http://who.int/biologicals/areas/vaccines/INFLUENZA_WG_mtg_TRS941_Annex_5_12_Oct_2017_for_web.pdf?ua=1, accessed 22 January 2019).

9. Informal consultation on WHO biosafety risk assessment and guidelines for the production and quality control of novel human influenza candidate vaccine viruses and pandemic vaccines. Geneva, Switzerland, 23–24 April 2018. Geneva: World Health Organization; 2018 (http://www.who.int/biologicals/areas/vaccines/WHO_flu_meeting_(April_2018)_report_ver3_20181019-final.pdf?ua=1, accessed 22 January 2019).

10. Production of pilot lots of inactivated influenza vaccines from reassortants derived from avian influenza viruses. Interim biosafety risk assessment. Geneva: World Health Organization; 2003 (Document WHO/CDS/CSR/RMD/2003.5; http://www.who.int/csr/resources/publications/influenza/influenzaRMD2003_5.pdf, accessed 22 January 2019).

11. Laboratory biosafety manual. Third edition. Geneva: World Health Organization; 2004 (Document WHO/CDS/CSR/LYO/2004.11; https://www.who.int/csr/resources/publications/biosafety/Biosafety7.pdf?ua=1, accessed 22 January 2019).

12. Neumann G, Kawaoka Y. Transmission of influenza A viruses. Virology. 2015;479–480:234–46 (https://www.ncbi.nlm.nih.gov/pmc/articles/PMC4424116/, accessed 23 January 2019).

13. Böttcher-Friebertshäuser E, Garten W, Matrosovich M, Klenk HD. The hemagglutinin: a determinant of pathogenicity. In: Compans R, Oldstone M, editors. Influenza pathogenesis and control - Volume I. Curr Top Microbiol Immunol. 2014;385:3–34 (abstract: https://link.springer.com/chapter/10.1007%2F82_2014_384, accessed 23 January 2019).

14. Robertson JS, Engelhardt OG. Developing vaccines to combat pandemic influenza. Viruses. 2010;2(2):532–46 (https://www.ncbi.nlm.nih.gov/pmc/articles/PMC3185603/, accessed 23 January 2019).

15. Recommendations for the production and control of influenza vaccine (inactivated). In: WHO Expert Committee on Biological Standardization: fifty-fourth report. Geneva: World Health Organization; 2005: Annex 3 (WHO Technical Report Series, No. 927; http://www.who.int/biologicals/publications/trs/areas/vaccines/influenza/ANNEX%203%20InfluenzaP99-134.pdf?ua=1, accessed 23 January 2019).

16. Recommendations to assure the quality, safety and efficacy of influenza vaccines (human, live attenuated) for intranasal administration. In: WHO Expert Committee on Biological Standardization: sixtieth report. Geneva: World Health Organization; 2013: Annex 4 (WHO Technical Report Series, No. 977; http://www.who.int/biologicals/areas/vaccines/influenza/TRS_977_Annex_4.pdf?ua=1, accessed 23 January 2019).

17. Rudenko L, Yeolekar L, Kiseleva I, Isakova-Sivak I. Development and approval of live attenuated influenza vaccines based on Russian master donor viruses: process challenges and success stories. Vaccine. 2016;34(45):5436–41 (https://www.sciencedirect.com/science/article/pii/S0264410X16306752, accessed 23 January 2019).

18. Guidance on regulations for the transport of infectious substances 2017–2018. Geneva: World Health Organization; 2017 (Document WHO/WHE/CPI/2017.8; http://apps.who.int/iris/bitstream/handle/10665/254788/WHO-WHE-CPI-2017.8-eng.pdf?sequence=1, accessed 23 January 2019).

19. Pandemic influenza risk management. A WHO guide to inform & harmonize national & international pandemic preparedness and response. Geneva: World Health Organization; 2017 (Document WHO/WHE/IHM/GIP/2017.1; https://apps.who.int/iris/bitstream/handle/10665/259893/WHO-WHE-IHM-GIP-2017.1-eng.pdf;jsessionid=91D4CE2B48055D403ECF6A5F8FB5CF50?sequence=1, accessed 8 February 2019).

20. Guideline on influenza vaccines. Non-clinical and clinical module. Committee for Medicinal Products for Human Use, 21 July 2016. London: European Medicines Agency. (Document EMA/CHMP/VWP/457259/2014; http://www.ema.europa.eu/docs/en_GB/document_library/Scientific_guideline/2016/07/WC500211324.pdf, accessed 23 January 2019).

21. Tripp RA, Tompkins SM. Virus-vectored influenza virus vaccines. Viruses. 2014;6(8):3055–79 (https://www.ncbi.nlm.nih.gov/pmc/articles/PMC4147686/, accessed 23 January 2019).

22. Lambe T. Novel viral vectored vaccines for the prevention of influenza. Mol Med. 2012;18(1):1153–60 (https://www.ncbi.nlm.nih.gov/pmc/articles/PMC3510293/, accessed 23 January 2019).

23. Wohlbold TJ, Krammer F. In the shadow of hemagglutinin: a growing interest in influenza viral neuraminidase and its role as a vaccine antigen. Viruses. 2014;6(6):2465–94 (https://www.ncbi.nlm.nih.gov/pmc/articles/PMC4074938/, accessed 23 January 2019).

24. Engelhardt OG. Many ways to make an influenza virus – review of influenza virus reverse genetics methods. Influenza Other Respir Viruses. 2013;7(3):249–56 (https://onlinelibrary.wiley.com/doi/full/10.1111/j.1750-2659.2012.00392.x, accessed 23 January 2019).

25. Garten W, Bosch FX, Linder D, Rott R, Klenk H-D. Proteolytic activation of the influenza virus hemagglutinin: the structure of the cleavage site and the enzymes involved in cleavage. Virology. 1981;115(2):361–74 (abstract: https://www.sciencedirect.com/science/article/abs/pii/0042682281901173, accessed 23 January 2019).

26. Dormitzer PR, Suphaphiphat P, Gibson DG, Wentworth DE, Stockwell TB, Algire MA et al. Synthetic generation of influenza vaccine viruses for rapid response to pandemics. Sci Transl Med. 2013;5(185):185ra68 (abstract: https://www.ncbi.nlm.nih.gov/pubmed/23677594, accessed 23 January 2019).

27. Fulvini AA, Ramanunninair M, Le J, Pokorny BA, Arroyo JM, Silverman J et al. Gene constellation of influenza A virus reassortants with high growth phenotype prepared as seed candidates for vaccine production. PLoS One. 2011;6(6):e20823 (https://www.ncbi.nlm.nih.gov/pmc/articles/PMC3113853/, accessed 23 January 2019).

28. Verity EE, Camuglia S, Agius CT, Ong C, Shaw R, Barr I et al. Rapid generation of pandemic influenza virus vaccine candidate strains using synthetic DNA. Influenza Other Respir Viruses. 2012;6(2):101–9 (https://www.ncbi.nlm.nih.gov/pmc/articles/PMC4942080/, accessed 23 January 2019).

29. Robertson JS, Nicolson C, Newman R, Major D, Dunleavy U, Wood JM. High growth reassortant influenza vaccine viruses: new approaches to their control. Biologicals. 1992;20(3):213–20 (abstract: https://www.ncbi.nlm.nih.gov/pubmed/1457106, accessed 23 January 2019).

30. Kilbourne ED. Future influenza vaccines and the use of genetic recombinants. Bull World Health Organ. 1969;41:643–5 (https://www.ncbi.nlm.nih.gov/pmc/articles/PMC2427719/pdf/bullwho00220-0293.pdf, accessed 23 January 2019).

31. Kilbourne ED, Schulman JL, Schild GC, Schloer G, Swanson J, Bucher D. Correlated studies of a recombinant influenza-virus vaccine. I. Derivation and characterization of virus and vaccine. J Infect Dis. 1971;124(5):449–62 (abstract: https://academic.oup.com/jid/article-abstract/124/5/449/913760?redirectedFrom=fulltext, accessed 23 January 2019).

32. Beare AS, Hall TS. Recombinant influenza-A viruses as live vaccines for man: Report to the Medical Research Council's Committee on Influenza and other Respiratory Virus Vaccines. Lancet. 1971;298(7737):1271–3 (abstract: https://www.sciencedirect.com/science/article/pii/S0140673671905976, accessed 23 January 2019).

33. Beare AS, Schild GC, Craig JW. Trials in man with live recombinants made from A/PR/8/34 (H0 N1) and wild H3 N2 influenza viruses. Lancet. 1975;306(7938):729–32 (abstract: https://www.sciencedirect.com/science/article/pii/S0140673675907205, accessed 23 January 2019).

34. Coelingh KL, Luke CJ, Jin H, Talaat KR. Development of live attenuated influenza vaccines against pandemic influenza strains. Expert Rev Vaccines. 2014;13(7):855–71 (abstract: https://www.ncbi.nlm.nih.gov/pubmed/24867587, accessed 23 January 2019).

35. Rudenko L, Isakova-Sivak I. Pandemic preparedness with live attenuated influenza vaccines based on A/Leningrad/134/17/57 master donor virus. Expert Rev Vaccines. 2015:14(3):395–412 (abstract: https://www.researchgate.net/publication/270397316_Pandemic_preparedness_with_live_attenuated_influenza_vaccines_based_on_ALeningrad1341757_master_donor_virus, accessed 23 January 2019).

36. Chen GL, Subbarao K. Live attenuated vaccines for pandemic influenza. In: Compans R, Orenstein W, editors. Vaccines for pandemic influenza. Curr Top Microbiol Immunol. 2009; 333:109–32 (abstract: https://link.springer.com/chapter/10.1007%2F978-3-540-92165-3_5, accessed 23 January 2019).

37. Li Q, Zhou L, Zhou M, Chen Z, Li F, Wu H et al. Epidemiology of human infections with avian influenza A(H7N9) virus in China. N Engl J Med. 2014;370:520–32 (https://www.nejm.org/doi/pdf/10.1056/NEJMoa1304617, accessed 23 January 2019).

38. Nicolson C, Major D, Wood JM, Robertson JS. Generation of influenza vaccine viruses on Vero cells by reverse genetics: an H5N1 candidate vaccine strain produced under a quality system. Vaccine. 2005;23(22):2943–52 (abstract: https://www.ncbi.nlm.nih.gov/pubmed/15780743, accessed 24 January 2019).

39. Webby RJ, Perez DR, Coleman JS, Guan Y, Knight JH, Govorkova EA et al. Responsiveness to a pandemic alert: use of reverse genetics for rapid development of influenza vaccines. Lancet. 2004;363(9415):1099–103 (abstract: https://www.sciencedirect.com/science/article/pii/S0140673604158923, accessed 24 January 2019).

40. Sun X, Tse LV, Ferguson AD, Whittaker GR. Modifications to the hemagglutinin cleavage site control the virulence of a neurotropic H1N1 influenza virus. J Virol. 2010;84(17):8683–90 (https://www.ncbi.nlm.nih.gov/pmc/articles/PMC2919019/, accessed 24 January 2019).

41. Couceiro JNSS, Paulson JC, Baum LG. Influenza virus strains selectively recognize sialyloligosaccharides on human respiratory epithelium: the role of the host cell in selection of hemagglutinin receptor specificity. Virus Res. 1993;29(2):155–65 (abstract: https://www.researchgate.net/publication/14986137_Influenza_virus_strains_selectively_recognize_sialyloligosaccharides_on_human_respiratory_epithelium_the_role_of_the_host_cell_in_selection_of_hemagglutinin_receptor_specificity, accessed 24 January 2019).

42. Matrosovich MN, Matrosovich TY, Gray T, Roberts NA, Klenk H-D. Human and avian influenza viruses target different cell types in cultures of human airway epithelium. Proc Natl Acad Sci U S A. 2004;101(13):4620–4 (https://www.pnas.org/content/101/13/4620, accessed 24 January 2019).

43. Chen Y, Liang W, Yang S, Wu N, Gao H, Sheng J et al. Human infections with the emerging avian influenza A H7N9 virus from wet market poultry: clinical analysis and characterisation of viral genome. Lancet. 2013;381(9881):1916–25 (abstract: https://www.thelancet.com/pdfs/journals/lancet/PIIS0140-6736(13)60903-4.pdf, accessed 24 January 2019).

44. Xiong X, Xiao H, Martin SR, Coombs PJ, Liu J, Collins PJ et al. Enhanced human receptor binding by H5 haemagglutinins. Virology. 2014;456–457(100):179–87 (https://www.ncbi.nlm.nih.gov/pmc/articles/PMC4053833/, accessed 24 January 2019).

45. Watanabe Y, Ibrahim MS, Ellakany HF, Kawashita N, Mizuike R, Hiramatsu H et al. Acquisition of human-type receptor binding specificity by new H5N1 influenza virus sublineages during their emergence in birds in Egypt. PLoS Pathog. 2011;7(5):e1002068 (https://www.ncbi.nlm.nih.gov/pmc/articles/PMC3102706/, accessed 24 January 2019).

46. WHO guidance on development of influenza vaccine reference viruses by reverse genetics. Geneva: World Health Organization; 2005 (Document WHO/CDS/CSR/GIP/2005.6; https://www.who.int/csr/resources/publications/influenza/WHO_CDS_CSR_GIP_2005_6.pdf, accessed 24 January 2019).

47. Hatta M, Gao P, Halfmann P, Kawaoka Y. Molecular basis for high virulence of Hong Kong H5N1 influenza A viruses. Science. 2001;293(5536):1840–2 (abstract: https://www.ncbi.nlm.nih.gov/pubmed/11546875, accessed 24 January 2019).

48. Govorkova EA, Rehg JE, Krauss S, Yen H-L, Guan Y, Peiris M et al. Lethality to ferrets of H5N1 influenza viruses isolated from humans and poultry in 2004. J Virol. 2005;79(4):2191–8 (https://www.ncbi.nlm.nih.gov/pmc/articles/PMC546577/, accessed 24 January 2019). Erratum in J Virol. 2006;80(12):6195 (https://www.ncbi.nlm.nih.gov/pmc/articles/PMC1472583/, accessed 24 January 2019).

49. Wagner R, Matrosovich M, Klenk HD. Functional balance between haemagglutinin and neuraminidase in influenza virus infections. Rev Med Virol. 2002;12(3):159–66 (abstract: https://www.ncbi.nlm.nih.gov/pubmed/11987141, accessed 24 January 2019).

50. Gaymard A, Le Briand N, Frobert E, Lina B, Escuret V. Functional balance between neuraminidase and haemagglutinin in influenza viruses. Clin Microbiol Infect. 2016;22(12):975–83 (https://www.sciencedirect.com/science/article/pii/S1198743X16302312, accessed 24 January 2019).

51. Goto, H, Kawaoka Y. A novel mechanism for the acquisition of virulence by a human influenza A virus. Proc Natl Acad Sci U S A. 1998;95(17):10224–8 (https://www.ncbi.nlm.nih.gov/pmc/articles/PMC21489/, accessed 24 January 2019).

52. Tumpey TM, Basler CF, Aguilar PV, Zeng H, Solórzano A, Swayne DE et al. Characterization of the reconstructed 1918 Spanish influenza pandemic virus. Science. 2005;310(5745):77–80 (abstract: https://www.ncbi.nlm.nih.gov/pubmed/16210530, accessed 24 January 2019).

53. Beare AS, Webster RG. Replication of avian influenza viruses in humans. Arch Virol. 1991;119(1–2):37–42 (abstract: https://link.springer.com/article/10.1007%2FBF01314321, accessed 24 January 2019).

54. Belser JA, Katz JM, Tumpey TM. The ferret as a model organism to study influenza A virus infection. Dis Model Mech. 2011;4(5):575–9 (https://www.ncbi.nlm.nih.gov/pmc/articles/PMC 3180220/, accessed 24 January 2019).

55. Zitzow LA, Rowe T, Morken T, Shieh W-J, Zaki S, Katz JM. Pathogenesis of avian influenza A (H5N1) viruses in ferrets. J Virol. 2002;76(9):4420–9 (https://www.ncbi.nlm.nih.gov/pmc/articles/PMC155091/, accessed 24 January 2019).

56. Belser JA, Eckert AM, Tumpey TM, Maines TR. Complexities in ferret influenza virus pathogenesis and transmission models. Microbiol Mol Biol Rev. 2016;80(3):733–44 (https://mmbr.asm.org/content/80/3/733, accessed 24 January 2019).

57. Belser JA, Barclay W, Barr I, Fouchier RAM, Matsuyama R, Nishiura H et al. Ferrets as models for influenza virus transmission studies and pandemic risk assessments. Emerg Infect Dis. 2018; 24(6):965–71 (https://wwwnc.cdc.gov/eid/article/24/6/pdfs/17-2114.pdf, accessed 24 January 2019).

58. Manual of diagnostic tests and vaccines for terrestrial animals. Chapter 2.3.4. Avian influenza (infection with avian influenza viruses). Paris: World Organisation for Animal Health; 2015 (http://www.oie.int/fileadmin/Home/eng/Health_standards/tahm/2.03.04_AI.pdf, accessed 24 January 2019).

59. Szretter KJ, Balish AL, Katz JM. Influenza: propagation, quantification, and storage. Curr Protoc Microbiol. 2006 Dec; Chapter 15: Unit 15G.1 (abstract: https://www.ncbi.nlm.nih.gov/pubmed/18770580, accessed 24 January 2019).

60. Terrestrial animal health code. Chapter 10.4. Infection with avian influenza viruses. Paris: World Organisation for Animal Health; 2017 (http://www.oie.int/fileadmin/Home/eng/Health_standards/tahc/current/chapitre_avian_influenza_viruses.pdf, accessed 24 January 2019).

61. Robertson JS, Cook P, Attwell A-M, Williams SP. Replicative advantage in tissue culture of egg-adapted influenza virus over tissue-culture derived virus: implications for vaccine manufacture. Vaccine. 1995;13(16):1583–8 (abstract: https://www.sciencedirect.com/science/article/pii/0264 410X9500085F, accessed 24 January 2019).

62. Smith DB, Inglis SC. The mutation rate and variability of eukaryotic viruses: an analytical review. J Gen Virol. 1987;68(11):2729–40 (abstract: https://www.researchgate.net/publication/19838801_The_Mutation_Rate_and_Variability_of_Eukaryotic_Viruses_An_Analytical_Review, accessed 24 January 2019).

63. Swayne DE, Halvorson, DA. Influenza. In: Saif YM, Barnes HJ, Glisson JR, Fadly AM, McDougald LR, Swayne DE, editors. Diseases of poultry. Eleventh edition. Ames (IA): Iowa State University Press; 2003:135–60.

64. Keawcharoen J, Oraveerakul K, Kuiken T, Fouchier RAM, Amonsin A, Payungporn S et al. Avian influenza H5N1 in tigers and leopards. Emerg Infect Dis. 2004;10(12):2189–91 (https://www.ncbi.nlm.nih.gov/pmc/articles/PMC3323383/, accessed 24 January 2019).

65. Lee CT, Slavinski S, Schiff C, Merlino M, Daskalakis D, Liu D et al. Outbreak of influenza A(H7N2) among cats in an animal shelter with cat-to-human transmission – New York City, 2016. Clin Infect Dis. 2017;65(11):1927–9 (https://academic.oup.com/cid/article/65/11/1927/4049509, accessed 24 January 2019).

66. Pecoraro HL, Bennett S, Huyvaert KP, Spindel ME, Landolt GA. Epidemiology and ecology of H3N8 canine influenza viruses in US shelter dogs. J Vet Intern Med. 2014;28(2):311–8 (https://www.ncbi.nlm.nih.gov/pmc/articles/PMC4857996/, accessed 24 January 2019).

67. Subbarao K, Chen H, Swayne D, Mingay L, Fodor E, Brownlee G et al. Evaluation of a genetically modified reassortant H5N1 influenza A virus vaccine candidate generated by plasmid-based reverse genetics. Virology. 2003;305(1):192–200 (abstract: https://www.sciencedirect.com/science/article/pii/S0042682202917423, accessed 24 January 2019).

68. Ito T, Couceiro JNSS, Kelm S, Baum LG, Krauss S, Castrucci MR et al. Molecular basis for the generation in pigs of influenza A viruses with pandemic potential. J Virol. 1998;72(9):7367–73 (https://www.ncbi.nlm.nih.gov/pmc/articles/PMC109961/, accessed 24 January 2019).

69. WHO good manufacturing practices for biological products. In: WHO Expert Committee on Biological Standardization: sixty-sixth report. Geneva: World Health Organization; 2016: Annex 2 (WHO Technical Report Series, No. 999; http://www.who.int/entity/biologicals/areas/vaccines/Annex_2_WHO_Good_manufacturing_practices_for_biological_products.pdf?ua=1, accessed 24 January 2019).

70. Directive 2000/54/EC of the European Parliament and of the Council of 18 September 2000 on the protection of workers from risks related to exposure to biological agents at work. Official Journal of the European Union, L 262, 17/10/2000 P. 0021–0045. Brussels: European Agency for Safety and Health at Work (https://osha.europa.eu/en/legislation/directives/exposure-to-biological-agents/77, accessed 24 January 2019).

71. Lau LLH, Cowling BJ, Fang VJ, Chan K-H, Lau EHY, Lipsitch M et al. Viral shedding and clinical illness in naturally acquired influenza virus infections. J Infect Dis. 2010;201(10):1509–16 (https://academic.oup.com/jid/article/201/10/1509/992720, accessed 24 January 2019).

72. Biosafety in microbiological and biomedical laboratories. 5th edition. United States Department of Health and Human Services. 2009 (HHS Publication No (CDC) 21-1112; https://www.cdc.gov/labs/pdf/CDC-BiosafetyMicrobiologicalBiomedicalLaboratories-2009-P.PDF, accessed 24 January 2019).

Appendix 1

Testing for attenuation of influenza CVVs in ferrets

Laboratories testing for the attenuation of influenza CVVs in ferrets should make use of a panel of standard/reference viruses (referred to as "pathogenicity standards" in the following sections) with defined experimental outcomes for pathogenicity testing. The pathogenicity standards (to be established by WHO laboratories) serve as benchmarks for the pathogenicity test in ferrets and delineate the expected outcomes. The use of these standards will ensure that the attenuation of CVVs is being measured against common parameters independently of subtype. In order to be designated as attenuated, the CVV to be tested must show parameters of pathogenicity that are below the predefined values of a high pathogenicity standard and are in line with the values of an attenuation standard. Comparative attenuation with the parental wild-type virus is not necessary in this case. However, laboratories that have the capacity to evaluate the attenuation of a CVV compared with the parental wild-type virus can continue to do so. To minimize the expected experimental variability of results across different laboratories, the pathogenicity standards can be tested in ferrets at each testing laboratory according to the experimental protocol shown below when establishing the ferret model for pathogenicity testing and at regular intervals thereafter. The results of these tests should fall within the limits described for the pathogenicity standards. In cases of discrepancy, a review of the ferret model should be carried out and advice should be sought from experienced WHO laboratories.

Test virus

The 50% egg or tissue culture infectious dose (EID_{50} or $TCID_{50}$) or plaque-forming units (PFU) of the reassortant CVV or pathogenicity standard will be determined. The infectivity titres of viruses should be sufficiently high to allow infection with 10^6 to 10^7 EID_{50}, $TCID_{50}$ or PFU of virus and diluted not less than 1:10. Where possible, the pathogenic properties of the donor PR8 virus should be characterized thoroughly in each laboratory.

Laboratory facility

Animal studies with the CVV and the pathogenicity standards should be conducted in animal containment facilities in accordance with the proposed containment levels shown in Table A3.1 (see section 5 above). For untested CVVs, the containment level to be used for the ferret safety test is the one shown for the respective wild-type virus. In specific cases, such as for CVVs derived from synthetic DNA representing H5 and H7 HPAI viruses, the containment level may be lowered based on a virus-specific risk assessment. An appropriate occupational health policy should be in place.

Experimental procedure

Outbred ferrets 4–12 months of age that are serologically negative for currently circulating influenza A and B viruses and for the test virus strain are anaesthetized by either intramuscular administration of a mixture of sedatives – for example, ketamine (25 mg/kg) and xylazine (2 mg/kg) and atropine (0.05 mg/kg) – or by suitable inhalant anaesthetics. A standard virus dose of 10^7 to 10^6 EID_{50} (or $TCID_{50}$ or PFU) in 0.5–1 ml of phosphate-buffered saline is used to inoculate animals. The dose should be the same as that used for pathogenicity studies with the wild-type parental virus, if used, or the pathogenicity standards previously characterized and regularly assessed in the laboratory. The virus is slowly administered into the nares of the sedated animals, reducing the risk of virus being swallowed or expelled. A group of 4–6 ferrets should be inoculated. One group of 2–3 animals should be euthanized on day 3 or day 4 after inoculation and samples should be collected for estimation of virus replication from the following organs: spleen, intestine, lungs (samples from each lobe and pooled), brain (anterior and posterior sections sampled and pooled), olfactory bulb of the brain and nasal turbinates. If gross pathology demonstrates lung lesions similar to those observed in wild-type viruses or established standards, it is recommended that additional lung samples be collected and processed with haematoxylin and eosin staining for histopathological evaluation. The remaining brain tissue should be collected for histopathological evaluation in the event that infectious virus is detected in this tissue. The remaining animals are observed for clinical signs, which may include weight loss, lethargy (based on a previously published index) (*1*), respiratory and neurological signs, and increased body temperature. Collection of nasal washes from animals anaesthetized as indicated above should be performed to determine the level of virus replication in the upper airways on alternate days after inoculation for up to 7 days. At the termination of the experiment on day 14 after inoculation, a necropsy should be performed on at least two animals and organs should be collected. If signs of substantial gross pathology are observed (for example, lung lesions), the organ samples should be processed for histopathological evaluation as described above.

Expected outcome

Clinical signs of disease, such as lethargy and/or weight loss, should be within the predefined ranges of acceptable pathogenicity defined by the pathogenicity standards, and histopathology of the lungs should demonstrate attenuation when compared to wild-type viruses or established standards. Viral titres of the vaccine strain in respiratory samples should be within the ranges of acceptable virus replication defined by the pathogenicity standards. Replication of the CVV should be restricted to the respiratory tract. Virus isolation from the brain is not expected. However, detection of virus in the brain has been reported for some seasonal A(H3N2) viruses (*2*) where virus was detected in the olfactory bulb. Consequently, if virus is detected in the anterior or posterior regions of the brain (excluding the olfactory bulb) the significance of such a finding may be confirmed by performing immunohistochemistry to detect viral antigen and/or histopathological analysis of brain tissue collected on day 3 or day 4 and on day 14 after inoculation. The detection of viral antigen and/or neurological lesions in brain tissue would confirm virus replication in the brain. The presence of neurological signs and confirmatory viral antigen and/or histopathology in brain tissue would indicate a lack of suitable attenuation of the CVV.

A model summary table for reporting test results is provided in Table A3.A1.1 with the intention of harmonizing data reporting between laboratories testing for the attenuation of influenza CVVs in ferrets.

Table A3.A1.1

Summary of results in ferrets infected intranasally with CVV

Virus	Dose (EID$_{50}$)[a]	Number of animals	Number of animals with clinical signs to day 14 post-inoculation				Mean maximum % weight loss	Respiratory tract viral titres (log$_{10}$ EID$_{50}$/ml or TCID$_{50}$)[b]		Lung lesions (day 3/4)[c,d]	Lung lesions (day 14)[c,d]	Detection of virus in other organ[e]
			Lethargy	Respiratory	Weight loss	Other (e.g. fever)		Mean peak nasal wash or nasal turbinate	Lung			
CVV												
Reference virus(es)												

[a] Indicate whether dose is expressed as EID$_{50}$, TCID$_{50}$ or PFU.

[b] Indicate whether respiratory viral titres are expressed as EID$_{50}$, TCID$_{50}$ or PFU per ml or g. Give lower limit of detection.

[c] Score gross pathological lung lesions as: − (absent); + (≤ 20%); ++ (> 20% but < 70%); or +++ (> 70%).

[d] Indicate outcome of any histopathological evaluation.

[e] Indicate organ or not detected.

References

1. Reuman PD, Keely S, Schiff GM. Assessment of signs of influenza illness in the ferret model. J Virol Methods. 1989;24(1–2)27–34 (abstract: https://www.sciencedirect.com/science/article/pii/0166093489900049, accessed 6 February 2019).

2. Zitzow LA, Rowe T, Morken T, Shieh W-J, Zaki S, Katz JM. Pathogenesis of avian influenza A (H5N1) viruses in ferrets. J Virol. 2002;76(9):4420–9 (https://www.ncbi.nlm.nih.gov/pmc/articles/PMC155091/, accessed 6 February 2019).

Annex 4

Guidelines for the safe production and quality control of poliomyelitis vaccines

Replacement of Annex 2 of WHO Technical Report Series, No. 926

Guidelines published by the World Health Organization (WHO) are intended to be scientific and advisory in nature. Each of the following sections constitutes guidance for national regulatory authorities (NRA) and for manufacturers of poliomyelitis vaccines. If an NRA so desires, these WHO Guidelines may be adopted as definitive national requirements, or modifications may be justified and made by the NRA. National requirements should be consistent with GAPIII and the Containment Certification Scheme, and should ensure that the risks of reintroducing poliovirus into the community are no greater than would be the case if these WHO Guidelines are followed. This document also sets out a number of guiding principles that might usefully be considered by national authorities for containment (NACs).

Abbreviations

CAG	Containment Advisory Group
$CCID_{50}$	cell culture infectious dose 50%
CCS	Containment Certification Scheme
CD155	cluster of differentiation 155 (also known as the poliovirus receptor)
cVDPV	circulating vaccine-derived poliovirus
CWG	Containment Working Group
GAPIII	WHO Global Action Plan to minimize poliovirus facility-associated risk after type-specific eradication of wild polioviruses and sequential cessation of oral polio vaccine use
GCC	Global Commission for the Certification of the Eradication of Poliomyelitis (also known as the Global Certification Commission)
GMP	good manufacturing practice(s)
HEPA	high-efficiency particulate air
IPV	inactivated poliomyelitis vaccine
NAC	national authority for containment
NRA	national regulatory authority
OPV	oral poliomyelitis vaccine
PEESP	The *WHO Polio Eradication & Endgame Strategic Plan 2013–2018*
PEF	poliovirus-essential facility
VDPV	vaccine-derived poliovirus

1. Introduction

The WHO Guidelines for the safe production and quality control of inactivated poliomyelitis vaccine manufactured from wild polioviruses (*1*) were developed in 2003 as an addendum to the previous Recommendations for the production and control of poliomyelitis vaccine (inactivated) (*2*), and specify the measures to be taken to minimize the risk of accidental reintroduction of wild-type poliovirus from a vaccine manufacturing facility into the community after global certification of poliomyelitis eradication.

In response to subsequent developments in manufacture and the progress of the poliomyelitis eradication programme, revised WHO Recommendations for the production of inactivated poliomyelitis vaccine (IPV) (*3*) and oral poliomyelitis vaccine (OPV) (*4*) have recently been published. Both of these documents highlight the need for enhanced biorisk management in the production and control of poliomyelitis vaccines after eradication but do not provide detailed guidance on this aspect. Vaccine production must comply with current good manufacturing practices (GMP) requirements to ensure product quality (*5, 6*). WHO guidance on good manufacturing practices for biological products (*6*) specifically emphasizes that the production of poliomyelitis vaccines should also comply with the containment requirements outlined in the third revision of the WHO Global Action Plan to minimize poliovirus facility-associated risk after type-specific eradication of wild polioviruses and sequential cessation of oral polio vaccine use (GAPIII) (*7*) to ensure the protection of personnel and the environment.

However, none of the currently available guidelines and recommendations provides sufficient detail concerning strategies or approaches for satisfying the objectives of both current GMP and GAPIII. Furthermore, some of these documents were developed based on different conceptual frameworks and often use incongruent terminology. It was recognized that revision of the 2003 Guidelines (*1*) was required in order to provide explicit, concise and updated guidance on the biosafety aspects of poliomyelitis vaccine production consistent with current GMP. In October 2015 the need for such a revision was raised at the WHO Expert Committee on Biological Standardization (*8*) with subsequent progress reported upon. The Committee agreed with the conclusions reached and the proposals made and expressed its support for the revision process (*8, 9*).

2. Purpose and scope

These revised WHO Guidelines provide information and guidance to vaccine manufacturers and relevant national authorities on the biosafety measures required for poliomyelitis vaccine production and quality control during the final poliovirus containment stage (Phase III) as defined in GAPIII (*7*). The current document specifies the biosafety-related steps to be taken to minimize the risk of accidentally reintroducing poliovirus from a vaccine manufacturing facility into the community after global certification of poliomyelitis eradication, and should be read in conjunction with other relevant WHO guidance (*3–7, 10*). Detailed and specific guidance on biosecurity has been described in GAPIII (*7*) and other WHO documents (*11*), and is therefore not repeated in the current document. Poliomyelitis vaccine manufacturers should implement these biosecurity measures to reduce the likelihood of intentional release of poliovirus.

Currently there are three types of poliomyelitis vaccines: OPV made from Sabin strains, IPV made from wild-type strains and IPV made from Sabin strains. IPV derived from wild-type strains and OPV are conventional vaccines developed and introduced in the 1950s and 1960s respectively. Recently, Sabin IPV has been introduced in Japan and China. Manufacturers are also working on alternative versions of poliomyelitis vaccines, with a number of candidate vaccines now in different phases of nonclinical and clinical development. These include: (a) safer and more genetically stable strains of OPV; (b) IPV made from genetically modified strains with improved biological characteristics that may require less stringent biosafety and biosecurity measures; and (c) poliomyelitis vaccines prepared by novel biotechnology processes that do not require the cultivation of live virus (for example, vaccines based on virus-like particles).

The previous version of these WHO Guidelines (*1*) dealt with the safe production and quality control of IPV based specifically on wild-type strains. These revised Guidelines address the containment measures needed during the production and quality control of:

- IPV produced from wild-type poliovirus strains;
- IPV produced from the live attenuated vaccine (Sabin) strains used in the manufacture of OPV;
- OPV and IPV produced from novel safer strains developed by genetic manipulation.

The document also covers the preparation of all viruses and other biological materials used in poliomyelitis vaccine manufacture and critical quality control tests. The production of poliomyelitis vaccines using platforms involving genetic expression systems without virus replication is outside the scope of these current Guidelines. However, any quality control test using live poliovirus should be carried out in a containment facility following the guidance provided by GAPIII and this document, unless the quality control procedures involve the use of safer virus strains approved by the WHO Containment Advisory Group (CAG) for handling outside of GAPIII containment (*12*).

The global eradication of wild-type 2 virus was declared in September 2015 (see section 3 below). The use of trivalent OPV then ceased with the withdrawal of the type-2 component in April 2016 and a global switch to bivalent OPV took place. The handling and storage of all type-2 poliovirus materials should now follow the guidance set out in GAPIII (*7*) and associated GAPIII Containment Certification Scheme (CCS) (*13*). Furthermore, the global cessation of OPV use is planned to take place after the declaration of wild-type poliovirus eradication, and OPV will only be used to respond to outbreaks of wild-type poliovirus or vaccine-derived poliovirus (VDPV). As a result, OPV prepared from Sabin strains is also outside the scope of this document (*9*).

3. Background

In 1988 the Forty-first World Health Assembly adopted a resolution (WHA41.28) to eradicate poliomyelitis by the year 2000 (*14*). Although the target date had subsequently to be revised, the number of cases and number of countries with poliomyelitis cases have both fallen drastically. There are three serotypes of poliovirus (1, 2 and 3). Wild-type 2 poliovirus has not been isolated since 1999, and was officially declared eradicated by the Global Commission for the Certification of the Eradication of Poliomyelitis (GCC) in September 2015. The last case of poliomyelitis caused by a wild-type 3 strain occurred in Nigeria on 10 November 2012. To date, wild-type 1 poliovirus remains endemic in several countries. Confirmation of the absence of poliovirus in circulation requires a prolonged period of intense surveillance as these viruses can circulate undetected for several years. This was recently illustrated by two cases of poliomyelitis caused by wild-type 1 poliovirus reported in Nigeria in August 2016. Since 2012 Nigeria had been considered to be free of wild-type polioviruses. In addition, the continued emergence of neurovirulent VDPVs necessitates the replacement of OPV with inactivated vaccines and/or with new further attenuated vaccines requiring appropriate characterization and clinical study to demonstrate their improved safety profile compared to current OPV. A number of efforts are under way to develop and introduce new vaccine products suitable for post-eradication vaccination programmes.

It is clear that if one country still has circulating poliovirus the world is at risk of reintroduction. This makes the containment of polioviruses during vaccine production and control vital to prevent their release into the environment and the re-establishment of poliovirus circulation. In 2004 poliomyelitis vaccination was stopped in Nigeria as a result of misinformation about the vaccine, and poliovirus was reintroduced across much of Central Africa as a result. In addition, outbreaks also occurred in Yemen and Indonesia as the virus was exported from Nigeria during the Hajj. In the past, poliovirus was repeatedly introduced into Angola from northern India, and other importations have occurred including from Pakistan into China and from India into Kazakhstan, the Russian Federation, Tajikistan, Turkmenistan and Uzbekistan. More recently, poliovirus was exported from Pakistan to Egypt, Israel and the Syrian Arab Republic in apparently separate events.

The main tool used in the poliomyelitis eradication programme has been OPV, which has been shown to interrupt transmission by inducing effective intestinal immunity. Eradication has involved the use of OPV during National Immunization Days and other immunization activities which supplement routine programmes where the vaccine is given in association with other childhood vaccines. This strategy has proven to be highly effective in eliminating poliomyelitis in most of the places where it has been used.

The OPV strains replicate in the gut of the recipient and are shed, potentially infecting contacts. The infection of contacts by excreted vaccine virus boosts immunity in those already immunized. However, where vaccination coverage is suboptimal, it is possible for the OPV viruses to regain both transmissibility and neurovirulence, and to develop into circulating VDPVs (cVDPVs) leading to poliomyelitis outbreaks. This has occurred on numerous occasions and has led to two specific changes to immunization practices. Firstly, a switch from OPV to IPV for routine immunization was made starting in high-income countries and more recently expanded to many others. Secondly, as the majority of cVDPVs are derived from the type 2 Sabin strain, countries using trivalent OPV switched in April–May 2016 to bivalent OPV containing only types 1 and 3 Sabin strains (*15, 16*). Type 2 Sabin strain is also the most effective in generating immune response in vaccinees, and competes with the other vaccine serotypes thus reducing their effectiveness. Poliomyelitis was eliminated in India when monovalent OPV and bivalent OPV (containing types 1 and 3 but not type 2) were used. On rare occasions, OPV can cause chronic infection in immunodeficient individuals, with the type 2 component being the most common cause. As a risk-mitigation measure, immunization with bivalent OPV can be supplemented by the use of IPV. Eventually, following the eradication of any remaining circulating poliovirus, bivalent OPV usage will also be stopped and will be replaced by the exclusive use of IPV or alternative versions of poliomyelitis vaccines as described in section 2 of this document. If there is a need for an emergency response to a poliomyelitis outbreak following eradication then stockpiles of monovalent OPV will be released by the Director-General of WHO (*17*).

Once eradication is complete, live polioviruses should be contained or destroyed to prevent the reintroduction of the disease – a process begun in 2015 with the type 2 strains. Production of IPV requires the cultivation of large amounts of live poliovirus which is then inactivated to destroy its infectivity. No poliomyelitis outbreak has yet been caused by the release of virus from a production facility even though accidental releases of poliovirus from IPV production plants have been documented. Biosafety may depend on several factors, and designing and operating facilities in ways that minimize virus escape while following production practices that protect workers from infection will be crucially important. Other key elements include ensuring high levels of immunization against poliovirus among the population in countries hosting vaccine production facilities and ensuring that adequate sanitation and hygiene conditions (including sewerage systems) are in place.

The need for larger quantities of poliomyelitis vaccine at lower prices to satisfy global demand has encouraged the development of manufacturing capability in areas of the world with little previous experience of IPV manufacture, inadequate sewage systems and effluent treatment, and greater potential for poliovirus transmission. Hence, this strategy poses additional risks and one possible mitigation strategy would be to base vaccine production on the strains used in OPV production. Their use in eradication, lower infectivity and reduced ability to spread suggest that they should be safer for production. However, the occurrence of cVDPVs and vaccine-associated poliomyelitis cases demonstrate the capacity of OPV strains to revert to a wild-type phenotype. As a result, despite potentially contributing to increased safety, the use of such strains cannot be relied upon exclusively. There is clearly a need to recognize, quantify and mitigate the risks associated with all vaccine production platforms.

The *WHO Polio Eradication & Endgame Strategic Plan 2013–2018* (PEESP) (*18*) was published by the Global Polio Eradication Initiative. This document discussed and summarized the complex nature of the endgame of poliomyelitis eradication. The subsequently developed and published GAPIII aligns the safe handling and containment of infectious and potentially infectious poliovirus materials with the PEESP. Taken together, GAPIII (*7*) and the GAPIII CCS (*13*) provide a framework for the containment of polioviruses by describing the systems and actions required to contain all types of work with polioviruses following their eradication, and should be read in conjunction with these WHO Guidelines. Following the requirement for the containment of wild-type 2 polioviruses and subsequent switch away from the use of Sabin type 2 in 2016, a phased approach to containment is currently under way. At present, only bivalent OPV consisting of type 1 and 3 Sabin strains is used, with the potential use of monovalent Sabin OPV2 reserved for controlling any future outbreak situation (*7*).

The destruction of unneeded poliovirus materials and containment of the remaining poliovirus stocks will be important considerations in the decision of the GCC regarding the eradication status of individual regions and of the entire world. To coordinate and oversee containment certification, GCC is supported by the Containment Working Group (CWG). The GCC and CWG will work with national authorities for containment (NACs) to scrutinize their certification applications and reports submitted by the poliovirus-essential facilities (PEFs) to check compliance against GAPIII requirements as they seek to certify their respective PEFs. According to the GAPIII CCS (*13*), the responsibility for PEF containment certification rests with the NACs in coordination with the GCC. Initial certification will result in the issuance of a Certificate of Participation,

WHO Technical Report Series, No. 1016, 2019

potentially followed by an Interim Containment Certificate. However, all PEFs intending to retain polioviruses will ultimately require a full Certificate of Containment. The certification of manufacturing facilities as PEFs will be based on compliance with the provisions of GAPIII and all other relevant regulatory requirements, standards and guidelines, including this document.

In 2017, WHO established the Containment Advisory Group (CAG), which includes experts in biosafety, biosecurity, virology, vaccine production and other relevant areas, and which acts as an advisory body to the Director-General of WHO. CAG meets on a regular basis to review and provide guidance on issues that are not fully covered in GAPIII. NACs and vaccine manufacturers are encouraged to submit to CAG any questions or requests regarding GAPIII implementation. For example, GAPIII describes in detail containment measures for wild-type and Sabin strains of poliovirus, but safer genetically modified strains have recently been developed with limited or no pathogenicity and transmissibility. Such strains, developed using recombinant technology, have been shown to have a better safety profile in laboratory studies, relative to wild-type or Sabin polioviruses, particularly with respect to genetic stability and the ability to infect human subjects. Strains unable to infect humans would be entirely safe and have therefore been proposed for use in the manufacture of poliomyelitis vaccines, and for conducting quality control tests and epidemiological surveillance. These new strains were developed to facilitate the manufacture and quality control of poliomyelitis vaccines by eliminating the need for costly and laborious containment procedures. To determine the appropriate containment measures for working with such strains, CAG formed an Expert Support Group consisting of poliovirus experts who advise CAG on specific aspects of the pathogenicity and transmissibility of the new strains. Based on a review of the scientific evidence, CAG recommended that genetically stabilized S19 strains of poliovirus can be handled outside of the containment requirements of GAPIII for the purposes of vaccine production and quality control testing. This and other CAG recommendations are published on the WHO website.[14]

4. Terminology

The definitions given below apply to the terms as used in these WHO Guidelines. These terms may have different meaning in other contexts.

Aerosol: a dispersion of solid or liquid particles of microscopic size in a gaseous medium.

---

[14] See: http://polioeradication.org/tools-and-library/policy-reports/advisory-reports/containment-advisory-group/, accessed 29 November 2018.

Air balance: the necessity to keep air supply and exhaust systems in balance by means of measurements of static pressure, fan and motor performance, and air volumes.

Airlock: an enclosed space with two or more doors which is interposed between two or more rooms (for example, of differing classes of cleanliness) for the purpose of controlling the airflow between those rooms when they need to be entered. An airlock is designed for either people (personnel airlock) or goods (material airlock).

Biological safety cabinet: Class II and Class III cabinets that are designed to protect the operator, the laboratory environment and work materials from exposure to infectious aerosols and splashes that may be generated when manipulating materials containing infectious agents, such as primary cultures, stocks and diagnostic specimens. Class II cabinets for microbiological work are partially open-fronted enclosures with air drawn around the operator into the front grille and a downward laminar flow of HEPA-filtered air that provides product protection by minimizing the chance of cross-contamination along the work surfaces of the cabinet. Class III cabinets are gas-tight enclosures with a non-opening view window, allowing access into the cabinet through a dunk tank or double-door pass-through box that is decontaminated between uses. Both the supply and exhaust air are HEPA filtered or incinerated before discharge. Airflow is maintained under negative pressure.

Biorisk: the biosafety and biosecurity risk related to a biological agent or material (in this case, poliovirus).

Biosafety: the containment principles, technologies and practices used to ensure the prevention of unintentional exposure to, or accidental release of, pathogens and toxins.

Biosafety manual: a comprehensive document describing the physical and operational practices of the laboratory facility with particular reference to safe working with biological materials.

Cell-culture infectious dose 50% ($CCID_{50}$): the quantity of a live virus that when inoculated onto a number of susceptible cell cultures will infect 50% of the individual cultures.

Certification: a systematic and documented process to ensure that systems perform in accordance with available certification standards or applicable validation guidance.

Closed system: a process system with equipment designed and operated such that the product is not exposed to the room environment.

Containment: a system for the confining of microorganisms or organisms or other entities within a defined space with controlled access.

Contingency plan: documented procedures for future events or circumstances regarded as likely to occur.

WHO Technical Report Series, No. 1016, 2019

Cross-contamination: contamination of a starting material, intermediate product or finished product with another starting material or product during production.

Decontamination: a procedure that eliminates biological agents and toxins or reduces them to a safe level.

Disinfection: the process of reducing the number of microorganisms (but not usually bacterial spores) without necessarily killing or removing them all.

Eyewash station: a dedicated device supplying clean fluids for emergency cleansing of eyes contaminated with biological or chemical agents.

Facility: any laboratory or vaccine production unit owned or operated by any level of government, academic institution, corporation, company, partnership, society, association, firm, sole proprietorship or other legal entity.

Good manufacturing practice (GMP): a system which ensures that products are consistently produced and controlled to the quality standards appropriate to their intended use and as required by the marketing authorization.

High-efficiency particulate air (HEPA) filter: a filter capable of removing at least 99.97% of all particles with a mean aerodynamic diameter of 0.3 μm.

Inactivation: rendering an organism unviable or a virus non-infectious by the application of heat, chemicals or radiation, or by other means.

National authority for containment (NAC): the national authority responsible for GAPIII containment certification. NACs are nominated by the ministry of health or other designated national body or authority.

Penetrations: openings through walls, floors or ceilings to allow access for mechanical services.

Poliovirus-essential facility (PEF): a facility designated by the ministry of health or other designated national body or authority as serving critical national or international functions that involve the handling and storage of needed poliovirus materials post-eradication under the conditions set out in Annex 2 or 3 of GAPIII (*7*). According to GAPIII, facilities are required to hold a valid certificate to handle and store polioviruses beyond Phase I (*7*).

Production: the entire set of processes and procedures involved in making vaccines that includes the manufacture of vaccine substances and components, formulation, quality control and filling of final containers.

Respirator: a respiratory protective device, with an integral perimeter seal, valves and specialized filtration, used to protect the wearer from toxic fumes or particulates.

Risk assessment: a systematic process of organizing information to support a risk decision to be made within a risk-management process. Risk assessment consists of the identification of hazards and the analysis and evaluation of risks associated with exposure to those hazards.

Sharps: laboratory devices capable of cutting or puncturing skin (for example, needles, scissors and glassware).

Sabin strains: preparations of polioviruses of types 1, 2 and 3 derived by limited number of passages from stocks developed by Dr Albert Sabin (*19*) which retain attenuated properties as measured by biological and molecular markers.

Validation: the documented act of proving that any procedure, process, equipment, activity or system actually leads to the controlled process.

5. General considerations

The production of poliomyelitis vaccines should be carried out in accordance with WHO recommendations for the manufacture and control of IPV (*3*) and OPV (*4*), as well as the general requirements outlined in WHO good manufacturing practices for pharmaceutical products: main principles (*5*) and WHO good manufacturing practices for biological products (*6*). In addition, the design and operation of poliomyelitis vaccine manufacturing and testing facilities should comply with the poliovirus containment requirements outlined in GAPIII (*7*).[15] GAPIII describes the containment requirements and procedures developed to minimize the risks of accidental release of poliovirus into the community from laboratories or other facilities that handle or store poliovirus. However, it does not provide guidance on assessing the specific risks associated with poliomyelitis vaccine manufacture. The production of poliomyelitis vaccines from wild-type, Sabin and new genetically modified safer strains raises a set of issues that require additional clarification for proper alignment of the above documents with GAPIII. The specific containment requirements and procedures will depend on the biological characteristics of vaccine strains and production conditions, and should be assessed on a case-by-case basis.

Requirements described in GAPIII should be reconciled with the provisions of current GMP as they apply to the manufacture of poliomyelitis vaccines. Thus, the current document should be read in conjunction with other relevant WHO guidance such as GAPIII (*7*), CAG reports,[16] GMP for biologicals (*5, 6*), the GAPIII CCS (*13*) and WHO laboratory biosafety and biosecurity manuals (*10, 11*), as well as other relevant documentation and national regulations governing the manufacture and control of these products. Alternative approaches are acceptable if demonstrated to be equivalent and approved by the appropriate national authorities. Contingency plans should be put in place for dealing with potential accidents. In most countries, the regulation of GMP and biosafety are governed by different institutions. Close collaboration between such

---

[15] See: http://polioeradication.org/polio-today/preparing-for-a-polio-free-world/containment/containment-resources/, accessed 29 November 2018.

[16] See: http://polioeradication.org/tools-and-library/policy-reports/advisory-reports/containment-advisory-group/, accessed 29 November 2018.

institutions is particularly important to ensure that both product contamination and environmental contamination levels are controlled within acceptable limits.

6. Biosafety implementation within a production facility for IPV

A breach of containment of poliovirus used in a vaccine production or testing facility could occur in a variety of ways, including through contact with contaminated equipment, clothing, skin and hair, or inadequate decontamination and disposal of liquid effluents, air emissions and other waste. In addition, inappropriate manipulation with live poliovirus leading to the exposure of personnel by oral and other routes (for example, via nose or eye) can result in asymptomatic infection and shedding of virus for several weeks. The amount of poliovirus required to cause infection by the oral route is thought to be 1 $CCID_{50}$ for wild-type and approximately 10^{1-2} $CCID_{50}$ for attenuated strains (*20, 21*). In production facilities, viral culture fluid before concentration contains poliovirus in the order of 10^8 $CCID_{50}$ per ml and bulk concentrates 10^{12} $CCID_{50}$ per ml. Based on these assumptions biosafety procedures may reduce the risk of accidental infection of workers in the plant but cannot remove it altogether. Accidental release and transmission from the laboratory or vaccine production facility to the community is most likely to result from either equipment failure or human error (*22, 23*). The inadvertent transmission of poliovirus to an immediate contact by an infected vaccine production worker has been documented (*24*).

Although Sabin vaccine strains are considered to be less transmissible than the wild-type poliovirus they can establish infections in suboptimally immunized populations, as the existence of cVDPVs demonstrates. There is also the possibility that a failure to either adequately identify an emergency situation or manage the risk associated with it could lead to the release of infectious materials into the community. The provisions in this document seek to minimize the risk of such occurrences.

6.1   The poliomyelitis vaccine manufacturer should employ one or more biorisk management advisers and establish a biorisk management committee as described in GAPIII. The biorisk management adviser(s) should be knowledgeable in poliomyelitis vaccine production, current GMP and containment, and be independent of production and quality control in their reporting structure. Senior management has the ultimate responsibility to ensure that an effective biorisk management system is in place.

6.2   A detailed and comprehensive risk analysis should be conducted to identify possible sources of contamination of personnel or the environment that may arise from the production or testing of live poliomyelitis vaccine within the establishment. For each procedure or system this risk analysis should take into account the volume, concentration and stability of the poliovirus at the site, the potential for inhalation, ingestion or injection that could result from accidents, and the potential results of a major or minor system failure. The procedural and technical measures to be taken to reduce the risk to workers and the environment should be considered as part of this analysis. The analysis should be documented and lead to the implementation of appropriate risk-mitigation strategies.

6.3   The biosafety aspects of the production process and quality control activities – including but not limited to response to biosafety emergencies and accidents, waste disposal and the requirements for safe practices and procedures as identified in the risk analysis – should also be documented, and reviewed and updated following a predetermined schedule.

7. Personnel

7.1   Personnel required to work in the poliovirus containment facilities, both manufacturing and testing, should be selected with care to ensure that they may be relied upon to observe the appropriate codes of practice, and are not subject to any disease or condition that could compromise the integrity of the product or the containment of the poliovirus strains with which they work. Acceptance by staff that adhering to biorisk management policies and procedures is an individual responsibility is a key factor in its implementation and maintenance, as described in GAPIII (7).

7.2   Procedures should be in place to ensure that all staff working at the containment facilities are of suitable health status before the start of employment and periodically thereafter following a predetermined schedule. Any changes in health status that could adversely affect the quality of the product or the containment procedures (for example, immune deficiency) should preclude the person concerned from working in the production or containment facilities.

7.3   Personnel working in poliovirus containment facilities should be immunized with poliomyelitis vaccines, and adequate blood titres of circulating neutralizing antibodies against all three serotypes should be confirmed, prior to their authorization to enter the containment facilities unless it is decontaminated following a validated process. The antibody titres should be monitored and a booster immunization given as needed. Temporary workers, contractors and visitors should also have protective immunity against poliovirus. Personnel entering the containment facilities only after decontamination of the facilities using a validated procedure may be exempted from the immunization requirement.

WHO Technical Report Series, No. 1016, 2019

7.4 All personnel (including those concerned with cleaning, maintenance or quality control) employed in containment facilities where live poliovirus is manufactured or tested should receive additional training and periodic retraining specific to their work with poliovirus. This should include relevant information and training in hygiene and microbiology in relation to poliomyelitis vaccine production and poliovirus, as well as biosafety procedures. Attention should also be given to ensuring that hygiene precautions are taken to minimize the risk of transmission of poliovirus from personnel to their family members and contacts.

7.5 **Personal protection:**

7.5.1 Personnel working in the containment facilities should be trained and deemed to be competent in all operating practices and standard microbiological practices – as outlined in the *WHO Laboratory biosafety manual (10)* – including gowning procedures and procedures for dealing with emergencies, biohazards and other hazards associated with the work.

7.5.2 Personnel should be provided with the facilities and equipment required to minimize potential exposure and to efficiently perform the required procedures. Efforts should also be made to ensure that the equipment provided to personnel is both ergonomic and comfortable. Provision should also be made for the changing of clothing and emergency decontamination of personnel in the event of a spill or other release of infectious materials.

7.5.3 Appropriate protective clothing and equipment should be provided based on risk assessment. For example, solid-front or wrap-around gowns, scrub suits or coveralls with head and shoe covers should be worn at all times by operators while in the containment facility. The use of eye protection or full-face masks should be required when there is a potential for generating aerosols. Respirators should be used when conducting procedures with a high probability of aerosol generation. Protective clothing is to be removed when leaving the containment facility, and should be decontaminated using a validated procedure before re-use or disposal.

7.5.4 Double gloves should be worn at all times in the containment facility and discarded as waste for decontamination in the dirty area of the personnel exit airlock. Outer gloves should be removed and discarded after handling potentially infectious materials.

7.5.5   Hands should be disinfected and washed upon leaving the containment facility. Hand-washing sinks equipped with automatic (hands-free) controls should be installed in the personnel exit airlock. All sinks should be connected to a validated waste decontamination system. The use of validated water-free (chemical) hand-washing systems with decontamination features is an acceptable alternative.

- Poliovirus is known to be resistant to many common disinfectants (*25, 26*). However, a recent study has shown that ethanol combined with 2-propanol, citric acid and urea is effective against poliovirus (*27*).

7.5.6   A full-body shower should be available within the personnel exit airlock from the containment facility. The use of a shower upon exit should follow the policies established by GAPIII and CAG[17] (*28, 29*).

7.5.7   Eyewash stations should be available, and their types and locations (for example, in a personnel airlock) determined by a risk assessment.

7.5.8   Good microbiological techniques should be followed (*10*). These include but are not limited to:

- no eating, drinking, smoking or applying of cosmetics in the containment facility;
- no mouth pipetting;
- implementing measures to minimize aerosol generation when manually transferring or mixing materials containing live poliovirus;
- implementing policies on the safe handling of sharps;
- conducting all manipulations of materials containing poliovirus under conditions of primary containment;
- decontaminating work surfaces after handling materials containing live poliovirus and after any spill of viable material; and
- decontaminating equipment before removing it from the facility for repair or maintenance.

---

[17] See: http://polioeradication.org/tools-and-library/policy-reports/advisory-reports/containment-advisory-group/, accessed 29 November 2018.

8. Premises and equipment

Premises should be designed in such a way as to control the risks to the product, the personnel and the environment. This is accomplished by using appropriate primary containment devices such as biological safety cabinets, isolators, vessels and transfer pipes to protect personnel and the immediate workspace within the containment facilities, and by segregating the containment facilities with physical barriers, effluent treatments, airlocks and pressure differentials that protect the environment external to them from accidental exposure to infectious materials. These systems should also provide adequate safeguards to protect the product against contamination with extraneous agents and to prevent the cross-contamination of intermediates that have undergone viral inactivation.

8.1 **General requirements:**

8.1.1 Live poliovirus and materials in which live poliovirus may be present should be handled in contained areas. Contaminated materials, including equipment for repair or maintenance, should be decontaminated by a validated method prior to removal from the containment facility.

8.1.2 Whenever possible, poliomyelitis vaccine production facilities where live poliovirus is processed should be housed in dedicated buildings. If they are located in multipurpose buildings then the dedicated production facility should be separated by a physical barrier, and should have separate entrances and exits, dedicated effluent treatment systems and a dedicated ventilation system. Poliomyelitis vaccine quality control laboratories located in multipurpose buildings should be equipped with dedicated air handling and waste disposal systems that prevent the contamination of other areas with material infected with poliovirus.

8.1.3 Use of the poliovirus facility for the production of other microorganisms on a campaign basis may be acceptable provided that a changeover procedure is validated and implemented as outlined in Annexes 2 and 3 of GAPIII.

8.1.4 All containment facilities where live poliovirus is stored, handled and treated should be marked with approved biohazard signs. Signs should be posted in prominent locations at the entry to the facility clearly stating that poliovirus is contained in the area and that only personnel authorized to work with poliovirus are permitted to enter. The name(s) and contact information of persons to be contacted in the event of an emergency should be displayed at all times and kept up to date.

8.1.5 All exits should be marked. Emergency exit doors from the poliovirus facility should be alarmed and their use treated as a breach of containment unless a closed system is maintained for processes involving the use of viruses.

8.1.6 Vision panels may be used to allow visual monitoring of activities in the laboratory and production areas inside the containment facility. Other devices such as closed-circuit television cameras may be effective alternatives where vision panels are not appropriate.

8.2 Equipment:

8.2.1 Biological safety cabinets or equivalent equipment should be provided within the production and quality control areas, and should be used for procedures involving the handling or manipulation of live poliovirus or infected cell cultures.

8.2.2 Biological safety cabinets should be constructed and manufactured in accordance with national regulations or standards, such as EN 12469, British Standards Institution (BSI), Deutsche Industries Norm (DIN) or National Sanitation Foundation (NSF). They should be tested and certified on a regular schedule as meeting those standards. Cabinets with design modifications to meet the requirements of large-scale operations, but providing equivalent containment levels, may be used if approved by the responsible national authorities and if they also meet the manufacturer's specifications.

8.2.3 When exhaust air from biological safety cabinets is to be discharged through the building exhaust air system, the air handling system should be designed in such a way as to not disturb the air balance of the cabinet or of the room in which the cabinet is situated.

8.2.4 Whenever possible, manufacturing process and transfer of intermediates should be carried out in closed systems.

8.2.5 In situations where production failure, product contamination or similar reason necessitates the discarding of a batch, there should be a predetermined and validated procedure for inactivating the contents of the full tank/container. This procedure should be described in sufficient detail and all relevant staff should be trained in it with such training documented.

8.2.6 All equipment used to handle and store live poliovirus should be designed and operated in such a manner as to prevent uncontrolled release through any potential route of entry and exit (for example, air exhausts, waste lines, etc.). Suitable measures for testing, as well as alarms, should also be incorporated into the design and operation of such equipment.

8.3 Production facilities:

All poliomyelitis vaccine manufacturing steps that involve the processing of live poliovirus, including viral culture, viral purification and viral inactivation (*3*), should be performed within the containment facility. The design of the containment facility should also permit the effective segregation of the live virus and inactivation stages to prevent cross-contamination, as required by current GMP.

8.3.1 Areas used for the storage of poliovirus seed stock should be fully secured against entry by non-authorized personnel. For secondary (back-up) seed storage locations where stocks are not normally used for production, the NRA may approve storage in leak-proof containment containers within a dedicated freezer that is subject to security and access restrictions appropriate for the storage of poliovirus. Outside the containment facility, polioviruses should be stored under appropriate containment conditions, as determined by a risk assessment approved by the competent authority (for example, the NAC) and in line with the approach detailed in the GAPIII CCS (*13*) as recommended by CAG (*30*).

- The viral seed stock should be inventoried. The addition or removal of material should only be undertaken by authorized personnel following the approval of two authorized signatories on record, or the electronic equivalent of this approval. Records of the addition or removal of viral seed should be securely stored.

- The viral seed storage area should be equipped with a back-up emergency power source and with recording and alarm systems to monitor freezers.

8.3.2 The air flow system of the containment facility (including personnel and material airlocks) should be designed to prevent a breach of virus containment. The containment facility should be appropriately designed to facilitate the maintenance of negative pressure relative to the environment and of the required pressure cascades as described in WHO good manufacturing practices for pharmaceutical products containing hazardous substances (*31*). Adequate measures should be in place to prevent cross-contamination within the containment facility – for example, the segregation of an area of higher contamination risk (for example, viral culture and purification area) from an area of lower contamination risk (for example, stage 2 inactivation area).

8.3.3　An air handling system should maintain a negative pressure (inward directional air flows) in areas where live poliovirus is handled or where there is a potential for room contamination (for example, spills).

- The installation of high-efficiency particulate air (HEPA) filters provides a filter efficiency of 99.97% or greater removal of 0.3 μm particles. According to EN 1822 specifications, a HEPA filter with a minimum rating of H13 should be used. Air from areas where live poliovirus is handled or where there is a potential for contamination should be extracted through HEPA filters at the point of air removal from the chamber or sealable ducts.

- HEPA-filtered exhaust air may be recirculated to the same poliovirus containment facility – as described in WHO good manufacturing practices for pharmaceutical products containing hazardous substances (*31*) and WHO Guidelines on heating, ventilation and air-conditioning systems for non-sterile pharmaceutical products (*32*). A proper system for the maintenance and testing of HEPA filters should be in place. An energy recovery wheel or alternative may be used if the potential for cross-contamination is adequately addressed as outlined in the above WHO guidelines (*31, 32*). HEPA filter housings should be designed to allow for in situ filter isolation, decontamination and testing. Such filters should be tested and certified upon installation and at least annually thereafter.

- Pressure differential monitoring lines penetrating the containment barrier should be provided with HEPA filtration or acceptable alternative. This is not required for containment facilities with sealable pressure differential monitoring devices.

- Pressure difference readings for rooms should be controlled and monitored to ensure continuous compliance with defined parameters, and records should be maintained. The limits defined should be justified as outlined in WHO guidelines (*32*). Appropriate air pressure alarm systems should be installed to warn of any pressure cascade reversal or loss of design pressure status. The appropriate design, alert and action limits should be set. System redundancies should also be in place to respond appropriately to pressure cascade failure as outlined in WHO guidelines (*31*).

- Supply and exhaust air systems should be provided with automatic mechanical/electronic interlocks or other appropriate devices that prevent sustained positive pressurization of the containment facility (*31*). The heating, ventilation and air conditioning (HVAC) system and controls should be verified during scenarios simulating the failure of system components, including exhaust fan(s), supply fan(s), power and Class II B2 biological safety cabinet exhaust fan(s) (where present), as determined by containment facility design (*31*). The rate of removal of exhaust air should result in sufficient air changes in both the production and quality control areas to provide an appropriate level of environmental cleanliness.

8.3.4 The containment facility should have the following physical characteristics:

- Surfaces and interior coatings within the containment facility – including, but not limited to, floors, ceilings, walls, doors, frames, casework, benchtops and furniture – should permit easy and effective cleaning and decontamination, and should be non-absorbent and resistant to scratches, stains, moisture, chemicals, heat, impact, repeated decontamination and high-pressure washing.

- The design of the facility should incorporate hands-free controls where possible to avoid cross-contamination. For example, pull strings for opening airlocks, light switches, intercoms and faucets can all be replaced by elbow switches or motion detectors. A risk assessment should identify all potential sources of such cross-contamination and define a strategy to minimize these.

- There should be no window that can be opened or any direct venting opening to the outside. Vision panels should be constructed of break-resistant safety glass with strength characteristics conforming to those required for the purpose for which they are used.

- Passageways for pipes, tubes and ducts passing through the wall between the containment facility and surrounding areas should be completely sealed with materials resistant to contaminants and capable of withstanding disinfectants.

- Floor drains, where installed, should be capped, fitted with liquid-tight gaskets or connected to a waste effluent decontamination system to prevent inadvertent release into the sanitary drain.

- Provisions should be made to contain liquids leaking from bioreactors or tanks (including waste tanks) for a volume calculated as a worst-case scenario in relation to piping associated with the tanks and the media/water volumes through these systems that could contribute to the actual final spill volume.

- Liquid and gas services to the containment facility in which backflow may occur should be protected to prevent it. Vacuum lines should be protected with liquid disinfectant traps or HEPA filters or their equivalent.

8.3.5 If circulating water (for example, Purified Water or Water for Injection) is supplied in the containment facilities then the water treatment, storage and distribution systems should be designed, constructed and maintained with features for microbial control as described in WHO good manufacturing practices: water for pharmaceutical use (*33*). The method selected for microbial control should also be effective for inactivating poliovirus (for example, elevated temperature). An adequate monitoring system should be in place to ensure that the microbial control method works properly.

8.3.6 A communication system consistent with the facility containment conditions should be maintained between the containment facility and the support or administrative area to ensure safety and during emergencies such as spills. The communication system should be kept in working order at all times.

8.3.7 Emergency lighting and power to the containment facility and critical containment devices identified by risk assessment should be available.

8.3.8 In the event that any item is to be removed from the containment facilities it should be decontaminated as described in section 8.4 of this document or be sealed in an appropriate unbreakable leak-proof container (or containers) followed by a decontamination procedure to ensure that the exterior surfaces of the container(s) are free of infectious poliovirus.

8.4   **Decontamination and waste disposal systems:**

8.4.1   Decontamination of solid, liquid and gaseous wastes should take place within the containment facility.

8.4.2   The containment facility should be equipped with one or more interlocking double door pass-through autoclaves – the performance of each autoclave should be validated prior to its initial use and then periodically following a predetermined schedule. Autoclave condensate drains located outside the containment barrier should have a closed connection directly connected to the drain piping servicing areas inside the containment barrier, unless condensate is effectively decontaminated prior to release.

8.4.3   Decontamination technologies and processes should be validated prior to initial use and periodically revalidated following an established schedule and when significant changes to the processes are introduced.

8.4.4   Effluents from equipment, showers and sinks within the containment facility should be decontaminated by autoclaving or by discharge into a liquid effluent decontamination system. Such a system should be fully validated to ensure efficacy and be located in the containment facility. The effluent treatment tanks should be situated in an area with floor dams or other measures capable of containing the full tank volume and allowing for the full inactivation of its contents.

9. Documentation and validation

9.1   Detailed records of operating parameters for the containment facility should be produced and maintained for conducting assessments of facility performance.

9.2   All spills or accidental release of infected materials and the response to such events should be properly investigated and documented. The results of these investigations should be used to review and revise the applicable facility operating procedures.

9.3   The production facility and equipment should be designed and constructed in such a way as to allow for full validation and verification of containment processes. It is the responsibility of the poliomyelitis vaccine manufacturer to ensure that these facilities and equipment meet applicable standards and/or operating parameters that will ensure the containment of poliovirus as well as the protection of staff and the environment. Tests should be conducted following completion of facility construction or renovation. Regular maintenance should be carried out to ensure that the facility and equipment continue to meet the containment conditions. Records of the qualification and maintenance of the containment facility and equipment should be kept throughout the lifetime of the poliomyelitis vaccine production facility and for at least 5 years after the facility stops production. The containment features concerning biosafety to be assessed should include, but are not limited to, the following:

- integrity of containment perimeter, including penetrations through floors, walls and ceilings;
- integrity of the vessels, transfer pipes and other production equipment used to prevent the exposure of poliovirus to the room environment;
- sealable supply and exhaust ductwork between incoming and first outgoing HEPA filter ducting in the air handling system. The ducts should be considered to be part of the room up to the point of the disinfecting filter or incinerator;
- integrity of all HEPA and other high-efficiency filters and filter housings;
- directional inward air flow from non-contained areas to containment facility;
- biological safety cabinets and all primary containment devices;
- autoclaves for decontamination, including heat distribution and penetration studies, and biological challenge reduction studies if appropriate – validation studies should consider the worst case for load configurations;
- waste effluent systems and holding tanks;
- air, liquid and gas backflow prevention devices;
- alarm systems for air system failures, room pressure failures, electrical failures and failures of waste treatment systems;
- fire suppression devices and alarms; and
- communication systems.

9.4 Cleaning and disinfecting procedures should be validated and documented. Manufacturers are urged to develop and implement assays for monitoring the poliovirus on work surfaces. The data generated will facilitate biosafety management within the vaccine production and testing facilities.

9.5   Data sheets and associated materials that have been used in the containment facility should be decontaminated upon removal from the containment facility, or an electronic data gathering and transmission system implemented to transfer data from the containment facility.

10. Production

The production of poliomyelitis vaccine involves handling large volumes of concentrated live poliovirus within the containment facility. The operations are carried out using devices which are validated to maintain primary containment. Nevertheless, leaks can occur from valves or during procedures such as taking samples for testing purposes. Effective containment therefore requires that all aspects of production – from the specifications for the facility and equipment through to personnel and working procedures – be in compliance with GAPIII (*7*) and these WHO Guidelines.

10.1   The movement of all personnel involved in production and quality control testing should be controlled to avoid cross-contamination. In general, personnel should not pass from an area of higher contamination risk (for example, viral culture and purification area) to an area of lower contamination risk (for example, stage 2 inactivation area) within the containment facility per work day. If such movement is unavoidable, this should be managed based on the outcome of a risk assessment.

10.2 Material flow:

10.2.1   The flow of materials and equipment within the containment facility should be controlled to avoid cross-contamination.

10.2.2   Samples for quality control testing, and environment and water monitoring, should be sealed in appropriate unbreakable leak-proof containers and transported as described in section 8.3.8 above. If a disinfection procedure is used for the external container surfaces it should be validated and shown to have no impact on sample integrity. All samples should be handled safely and transported in accordance with applicable regulations.

10.2.3   Following a validated inactivation procedure, and prior to the confirmation of complete inactivation using a validated test approved by the NRA, the IPV monovalent bulk may be transferred out of the containment facility if the following conditions are met:

- The results of a battery of tests, which are predictive of complete inactivation, comply with the predetermined specifications. The battery of tests should include formaldehyde content and poliovirus loads at one or more time points during the inactivation. The integrity of the 0.2 μm filters used to remove aggregates at the beginning and middle of the inactivation process is critical and should be confirmed by testing at least post-use.

- A formal risk assessment is performed to estimate the likelihood of the occurrence of an incomplete inactivation, as well as the residual virus level in the case of an incomplete inactivation. Precautionary measures may be recommended based on the outcome of the assessment.

- A procedure is in place at the manufacturing facility to quarantine the IPV monovalent bulk transferred out of the containment facility until the completion of all quality control testing recommended in the WHO Recommendations to assure the quality, safety and efficacy of poliomyelitis vaccines (inactivated) (3), including the test for complete inactivation of poliovirus.

11. Quality control

The risks from live poliovirus in testing facilities are different from those in the production facilities. Although the volumes of poliovirus are smaller than those in the production facilities there are many more manual manipulations of samples and infected cell cultures containing viable polioviruses in testing facilities. The risk assessment should reflect these important differences.

11.1 Quality control testing laboratories should maintain containment conditions for all areas where materials containing live poliovirus are manipulated. Nucleic acid extracted from poliovirus should be handled in accordance with the recommendations made by CAG (28).

11.2 The quality control laboratories under containment conditions should be either poliovirus dedicated or used on a campaign basis using validated decontamination procedures in accordance with the recommendations made by CAG (28).

11.3 If quality control laboratories are housed within the production facility to enhance containment control then they should be kept separate from

WHO Technical Report Series, No. 1016, 2019

the production rooms, with separate air handling systems and dedicated airlocks for personnel and material provided from access corridors.

11.4 Quality control laboratories for poliovirus should be equipped with facilities for hand washing and disinfection. If sinks are used, the waste water should be collected in a waste disposal tank and disinfected prior to disposal. The use of validated water-free (chemical) hand-washing systems with decontamination features is an acceptable alternative. All solid, liquid and gaseous waste materials from the containment laboratories should be decontaminated prior to disposal.

11.5 All samples received from the containment production facility should be handled using established procedures to prevent the release of live poliovirus. Procedures used to decontaminate sample containers or packaging materials should be validated and shown to have no impact on sample integrity. The packaging materials should be decontaminated prior to disposal. All samples received from the containment production facilities – with the exception described below in section 11.6 – should be tested in containment laboratories. All test procedures using reagents containing live poliovirus should also be performed within the containment laboratories.

11.6 The Absence of Infective Poliovirus Test performed on the IPV monovalent bulk (*3*) – when transferred out of the containment production facility as described in section 10.2.2 above – may be performed outside the containment laboratories (*28*). However, the positive control of the test – along with the steps performed to demonstrate the sensitivity of the cells – require the use of live poliovirus and should be performed within the containment laboratories.

11.6.1 If the Absence of Infective Poliovirus Test is performed within the containment laboratories, care should be taken to prevent cross-contamination from the live poliovirus handled in the same area. If infective poliovirus is detected in this test, then extensive investigation is required – which will interrupt routine manufacturing and product release.

11.7 Test procedures involving the inoculation of animals with live poliovirus (such as neurovirulence tests) should be performed within containment laboratories and special care taken in line with GAPIII recommendations. Species susceptible to poliovirus infection, including transgenic mice expressing the human poliovirus receptor, should be treated as infectious materials following infection with virus samples. Non-susceptible animals inoculated with live poliovirus should also be considered as potentially infectious materials. This affects all aspects of work (including handling, transporting, storage, inventory, etc.) and also includes all animal-derived materials (including tissues, blood, carcasses, stools, etc.). The risk of infected animals escaping the facility should be assessed and managed as this represents a potential threat to the community. An animal-care manager should be designated with responsibilities conforming to the requirements of applicable national laws and as set out in these WHO Guidelines and other relevant documents. The animal-care manager should have an in-depth knowledge of animal handling, as well as of zoonotic and animal diseases. The animal-care manager should liaise with relevant personnel (for example, biorisk management adviser and occupational health professional) to implement effective and proportionate laboratory biosafety and biosecurity measures. A qualified veterinarian should be available for additional advice. The role should include providing input into risk assessment and management from an animal-care perspective. The poliovirus animal facility should incorporate features based on risk assessments and should accord with all poliovirus containment principles set out in this document.

12. Emergency procedures

Production and quality control testing of poliomyelitis vaccine using live polioviruses under containment conditions require planning for and practising emergency scenarios that could result in the release of live poliovirus within the facility or into the surrounding environment. The failure of containment systems within the facility as well as external events not under the control of the manufacturer could result in the exposure of plant personnel or the public to infectious poliovirus. Emergency response and contingency plans should be established based on risk assessment and should comply with the requirements outlined in GAPIII to minimize the impact and consequences of such incidents. These plans should be developed in collaboration with relevant first responder units. A memorandum of understanding and similar documents should be generated with a specific focus placed on conducting practice sessions with all relevant stakeholders present.

12.1 The response to an uncontrolled release of poliovirus resulting from a failure in containment systems should be planned and rapidly implemented to limit the exposure of persons to poliovirus.

12.1.1 The immediate response to a spill due to equipment failure (such as failure of vessels or transfer pipes) should be to stop the spill if possible and evacuate the premises, followed by the deployment of clean-up personnel no sooner than 30 minutes after the incident to allow time for any aerosols to settle.

12.1.2 Staff and emergency personnel should be supplied with protective equipment (for example, respirators, coveralls and gloves) prior to re-entering containment facilities for production or quality control. This equipment should be available in sufficient quantities at the entrance to the containment facilities and kept in good working order, with personnel having received prior instruction in its use.

12.1.3 The response should also include actions to limit the volume and distribution of the spill (for example, through the use of dams, spill socks and so on), as well as the use of validated methods for the inactivation of poliovirus and decontamination.

12.2 Emergency equipment such as disinfectants and other clean-up materials for spills should be available in sufficient quantities for use in responding to the release of infected material equivalent to the maximum capacity of the facility.

12.3 Emergency personnel should be immunized against poliomyelitis and have adequate training to enable them to understand the need for the containment measures in place. Whenever these precautions are not possible, emergency personnel should be supplied with adequate protective clothing and equipment to reduce the risk of them becoming infected with poliovirus in the course of their duties. Such protective clothing and equipment should be adequately disinfected before removal from the containment facility.

12.4 Personnel in the containment facility at the time of the spill, emergency response personnel, law enforcement, equipment/systems experts, medical or fire-fighting personnel, and those involved in the risk assessment, clean-up and disinfection of the area, all present a risk for a further breach in containment and subsequent poliovirus dissemination into the environment. Appropriate medical evaluation, surveillance and treatment should be provided following spills. Infected or potentially infected personnel should be monitored.

12.5 A full evaluation should be carried out after any emergency involving a breach of containment. The incident and all aspects of the response to it should be fully investigated and documented, and revisions made to existing procedures, contingency plans and staff training as necessary to minimize the risk of a repeat incident.

12.6 Any spill or accident that results in a breach of containment, as well as any suspected or confirmed poliovirus infection occurring within or surrounding the containment facility, should be investigated and documented as described above in section 9.2. The institutional biorisk management committee should be notified without delay.

13. Risk assessment of new safer strains of poliovirus

The biosafety and containment measures described above and set out in GAPIII were developed based on well-known biological characteristics of wild-type and attenuated Sabin strains used in the manufacture and control of poliomyelitis vaccines – including their ability to induce disease and to be transmitted from person to person. Since attenuated polioviruses used for the production of OPV can revert to virulence and regain the ability to be transmitted and cause outbreaks of paralytic disease, these measures reduce risks but do not eliminate them completely. New strains have therefore been developed by genetic manipulation based on detailed knowledge of poliovirus biology, with the specific purpose of stabilizing their attenuated phenotype and limiting their ability to infect humans and spread among populations. These strains have now been proposed for use in the manufacturing of new genetically stable OPV and IPV, and for performing quality control tests, to minimize or eliminate the risks of restarting poliovirus circulation. The introduction of these strains would not only significantly mitigate the consequences of accidental release of poliovirus but could also simplify the handling of virus stocks, and ultimately reduce the cost of vaccine manufacture thus increasing vaccine supply.

The containment measures appropriate for the new strains should be defined based on risk analysis performed on a case-by-case basis. If proven to be considerably safer than attenuated Sabin strains then such strains could, following NAC approval, be handled under containment conditions less stringent than those described in these WHO Guidelines or in GAPIII. CAG along with its affiliated Expert Support Group will review and evaluate the available scientific evidence and risk assessment, and advise on the appropriate level of containment for each new strain and new process proposed for implementation in poliomyelitis vaccine production and quality control.

The evaluation may consider the following elements:

13.1 Vaccine manufacturers proposing to handle strains with reduced virulence and transmissibility under less stringent containment conditions should perform a risk analysis and present it for approval to the appropriate national authorities. Risk analysis should be based on the biological properties of the specific strain, the intended use and design of the facility in which it will be used, and the proposed handling procedures. The criteria for evaluation of new strains listed by CAG include neurovirulence, genetic stability to loss of attenuation, replicative fitness and transmissibility (*12*). Based on these criteria, CAG reviewed the scientific evidence and recommended that genetically stabilized S19 strains of poliovirus can be handled outside of the containment requirements of GAPIII for the purposes of vaccine production and quality control testing.

13.2 An evaluation of neurovirulence can be carried out based on known in vitro markers as well as on experiments in laboratory animals. Several molecular structures within the poliovirus genome (for example, in the internal ribosome entry site (IRES) element) have been shown to be good predictors of neurovirulence. Animal models that could be used to evaluate neurovirulence include primates (rhesus and cynomolgus macaques) and transgenic mice expressing human poliovirus receptor CD155 (*34, 35*). Validated tests in both animal models were recommended by the WHO Expert Committee on Biological Standardization for use in the lot release of OPV (*4*) and could also be used to demonstrate the superior safety of new poliovirus strains. Such tests should include attenuated Sabin strains as the benchmark.

Another marker indicative of neurovirulence is the ability of viruses to replicate at higher temperature. Attenuated strains tend to grow better at sub-physiological temperatures, while pathogenic strains can grow at temperatures of up to 40 °C. Viruses producing lower yields of live virus can be expected to exhibit lower pathogenicity and transmissibility (see section 13.4 below).

13.3 Genetic stability is an important indicator of the safety of vaccine strains because replication in vitro and in vivo usually leads to reversion of the attenuated phenotype and the regaining of virulent properties. Genetic stability can be evaluated by both biological and molecular methods. Biological methods include passage in vitro and in vivo followed by neurovirulence testing in transgenic mice or monkeys. The molecular approach is based upon the quantification of mutants accumulated during virus growth by using direct methods such as nucleotide sequencing, mutant analysis by polymerase chain reaction (PCR) and restriction enzyme cleavage (MAPREC), and deep sequencing (*36, 37*).

13.4 There are no validated tests for the transmissibility of poliovirus. However, it can be inferred from a number of indirect markers. Lower stability of virus particles in the environment, lower yield of infectious virus (including shedding by susceptible animals infected orally) and an inability to grow at higher temperatures can all indicate that virus transmission will likely be restricted. It is possible to develop virus derivatives unable to replicate in normal cells, but which could grow in engineered cell cultures expressing factors enabling virus replication. Such viruses (that cannot grow in vivo) can be expected to be highly safe.

13.5 Appropriate containment conditions should be selected based on the above properties to minimize the risk of accidental virus release into circulation. Polioviruses shown to have significantly lower or no virulence in susceptible animal models, to be genetically stable upon passage and capable of replication only in specially designed cell cultures could be handled under conditions less stringent than those described above for wild-type and Sabin strains.

Authors and acknowledgements

The preliminary draft of these WHO Guidelines was prepared by Ms A. Bonhomme, Public Health Agency of Canada, Canada; Dr K. Chumakov, United States Food and Drug Administration, the USA; Dr J. Martin, National Institute for Biological Standards and Control, the United Kingdom; Dr P. Minor, National Institute for Biological Standards and Control, the United Kingdom; Dr T. Wu, Health Canada, Canada; and Dr I. Shin and Dr D. Wood, World Health Organization, Switzerland. The preliminary draft was then discussed during the WHO First Working Group meeting on developing WHO Guidelines on the safe production of polio vaccines held in Geneva, Switzerland, 22–23 September 2016 and attended by: Dr A. Albores, La Comisión de Control Analítico y Ampliación de Cobertura – la Protección Contra Riesgos Sanitarios, Mexico; Dr E. Augagneur, Sanofi Pasteur, France (*International Federation of Pharmaceutical Manufacturers & Associations (IFPMA) representative*); Ms A. Bonhomme, Public Health Agency of Canada, Canada; Dr C. Borgne, Biological E. Limited (Nantes), France (*Developing Countries Vaccine Manufacturers Network (DCVMN) representative*); Ms R. Bose, Central Drugs Standard Control Organization, India; Dr S. Brown, Biological E. Limited (Nantes), France (*DCVMN representative*); Dr M. Cereghetti, GlaxoSmithKline, Belgium (*IFPMA representative*); Dr K. Chumakov, United States Food and Drug Administration, the USA; Mr J. Clercq, Bilthoven Biologicals BV, Netherlands; Dr R. Dhere, Serum Institute of India, India (*DCVMN representative*); Dr M. Duchene, Janssen Infectious Diseases & Vaccines, Netherlands (*IFPMA representative*); Dr S. Fakhrzadeh, Food and Drug Administration, the Islamic Republic of Iran; Dr A. Fauconnier, Federal agency for medicines and health Products, Belgium; Dr M. Gonzalez, La Comisión de Control Analítico y Ampliación de Cobertura – la Protección Contra Riesgos Sanitarios, Mexico; Dr J. Hanselaer,

Sanofi Pasteur, France (*IFPMA representative*); Dr P.J. Huntly, Riskren PTE Ltd, Singapore; Dr C. Ilonze, National Agency for Food and Drug Administration and Control, Nigeria; Dr Y. Jee, Korea Centers for Disease Control and Prevention, Republic of Korea; Ms S. Jeong, LG Life Sciences, Republic of Korea (*DCVMN representative*); Dr J. Kim, Ministry of Food and Drug Safety, Republic of Korea; Ms Y. Kim, LG Life Sciences, Republic of Korea (*DCVMN representative*); Dr I. Knott, GlaxoSmithKline, Belgium (*IFPMA representative*); Mr H. Lee, LG Life Sciences, Republic of Korea (*DCVMN representative*); Dr H. Leng, Medicines Control Council, South Africa; Dr C. Li, National Institutes for Food and Drug Control, China; Dr K. Mahmood, PATH, the USA; Dr J. Martin, National Institute for Biological Standards and Control, the United Kingdom; Dr P. Minor, National Institute for Biological Standards and Control, the United Kingdom; Mr P. Morgon, AJ Biologics, Denmark; Mr T. Okada, BIKEN, Japan; Dr V. Pithon, Agence nationale de sécurité du médicament et des produits de santé, France; Ms E. Riayati, National Agency of Drug and Food Control, Indonesia; Dr A. Rietveld, Health Care Inspectorate, the Netherlands; Ms I. Rudebeck, Statens Serum Institut, Denmark; Dr T. Satu, Takeda Pharmaceutical Company Limited, Japan (*IFPMA representative*); Dr J. Shin, Ministry of Food and Drug Safety, Republic of Korea; Mr Y. Someya, National Institute of Infectious Diseases, Japan; Dr K. Stittelaar, Viroclinics, the Netherlands; Mr T. Tatsumoto, BIKEN, Japan; Mr A. Thomas, AJ Biologics, Denmark; Mr D. Ugiyadi, PT Bio Farma, Indonesia (*DCVMN representative*); Mr M. Usman, PT Bio Farma, Indonesia (*DCVMN representative*); Dr C. Villumsen, Ministry of Health, Denmark; Dr R. Wagner, Paul-Ehrlich-Institut, Germany; Mr B. Wibisono, National Agency of Drug and Food Control, Indonesia; Dr T. Wu, Health Canada, Canada; Mr H. Yeo, LG Life Sciences, Republic of Korea (DCVMN representative); Dr W. Yuan, China Food and Drug Administration, China; and Dr M. Chafai, Dr M Alali, Dr N. Previsani, Dr M. Refaat, Dr I. Shin and Dr D. Wood, World Health Organization, Switzerland.

The first draft of these WHO Guidelines was then prepared by a WHO Drafting Group comprising Ms A. Bonhomme, Public Health Agency of Canada, Canada; Dr K. Chumakov, United States Food and Drug Administration, the USA; Dr J. Martin, National Institute for Biological Standards and Control, the United Kingdom; Dr P. Minor, National Institute for Biological Standards and Control, the United Kingdom; Dr T. Wu, Health Canada, Canada; and Dr I. Knezevic and Dr I. Shin, World Health Organization, Switzerland. Comments on the first draft were received during the WHO Second Working Group meeting on developing WHO Guidelines on the safe production of polio vaccines held in Geneva, Switzerland, 19–20 September 2017 and attended by: Dr A. Albores, La Comisión de Control Analítico y Ampliación de Cobertura – la Protección Contra Riesgos Sanitarios, Mexico; Dr E. Augagneur, Sanofi Pasteur, France (*IFPMA representative*); Ms A. Bonhomme, Public Health Agency of Canada,

Canada; Mrs X. Bouwstra-Vinken, Bilthoven Biologicals BV, Netherlands; Dr C. Breda, Biological E. Limited (Nantes), France (*DCVMN representative*); Dr M. Cereghetti, GlaxoSmithKline, Belgium (*IFPMA representative*); Dr K. Chumakov, United States Food and Drug Administration, the USA; Dr M. Duchene, Janssen Infectious Diseases & Vaccines, Netherlands (*IFPMA representative*); Dr S. Fakhrzadeh, Ministry of Health and Medical Education, the Islamic Republic of Iran; Dr A. Fauconnier, Federal agency for medicines and health products, Belgium; Dr E. Febrina, National Agency of Drug and Food Control, Indonesia; Mr J. Hanselaer, Sanofi Pasteur, France (*IFPMA representative*); Mr B-K. Hyun, LG Chem, Republic of Korea (*DCVMN representative*); Dr C. Ilonze, National Agency for Food and Drug Administration and Control, Nigeria; Mrs A. Janssen, Bilthoven Biologicals BV, Netherlands; Ms S-G. Jeong, LG Chem, Republic of Korea (*DCVMN representative*); Mr J-H. Joo, LG Chem, Republic of Korea (*DCVMN representative*); Ms H-S. Kim, LG Chem, Republic of Korea (*DCVMN representative*); Ms I. Knott, GlaxoSmithKline, Belgium (*IFPMA representative*); Mr H-J. Lee, LG Chem, Republic of Korea (*DCVMN representative*); Dr H. Leng, Medicines Control Council, South Africa; Ms J. Li, Kunming Institute, China (*DCVMN representative*); Dr Q. Li, Kunming Institute, China (*DCVMN representative*); Mr Z. Li, China National Biotec Group, China (*DCVMN representative*); Dr J. Lim, Ministry of Food and Drug Safety, Republic of Korea; Dr K. Mahmood, PATH, the USA; Dr A. Malkin, Chumakov Federal Scientific Center for Research and Development of Immune-and-Biological Products, Russian Federation; Dr J. Martin, National Institute for Biological Standards and Control, the United Kingdom; Dr W. Meng, Sinovac Biotech, China (*DCVMN representative*); Dr P. Minor, London, the United Kingdom; Dr S. Ochiai, BIKEN, Japan; Mr T. Okada, BIKEN, Japan; Dr V. Paradkar, Biological E. Limited, India (*DCVMN representative*); Dr V. Pithon, Agence nationale de sécurité du médicament et des produits de santé, France; Ms I. Rudebeck, AJ Vaccines, Denmark; Mr S. Sharma, Ministry of Health and Family Welfare, India; Dr S. Sharma, Panacea Biotec, India (*DCVMN representative*); Dr A. Sinyugina, Chumakov Federal Scientific Center for Research and Development of Immune-and-Biological Products, Russian Federation; Mr Y. Someya, National Institute of Infectious Diseases, Japan; Dr G. Stawski, Statens Serum Institut, Denmark; Dr K. Stittelaar, Rotterdam Science Tower, Netherlands; Mr M. Sun, Kunming Institute, China (*DCVMN representative*); Mr H. Thuis, Bilthoven Biologicals BV, Netherlands; Mr A. Thomas, AJ Vaccines, Denmark; Ms N. Thuy, Ministry of Health, Viet Nam; Mr D. Ugiyadi, PT Bio Farma, Indonesia (*DCVMN representative*); Dr R.K. Vats, Ministry of Health and Family Welfare, India; Dr R. Wagner, Paul-Ehrlich-Institut, Germany; Dr T. Wu, Health Canada, Canada; Mr S. Yoon, LG Chem, Republic of Korea (*DCVMN representative*); Mr G. Yu, China National Biotec Group, China (*DCVMN representative*); Mr X. Zhang, Beijing Minhai Biotechnology Co. Ltd, China (*DCVMN representative*); Dr H. Zheng,

Beijing Minhai Biotechnology Co. Ltd, China (*DCVMN representative*); and Dr J. Fournier-Caruana, Dr I. Knezevic, Dr N. Previsani and Dr I. Shin, World Health Organization, Switzerland.

The second draft of these Guidelines was prepared by a WHO Drafting Group comprising Ms A. Bonhomme, Public Health Agency of Canada, Canada; Dr K. Chumakov, United States Food and Drug Administration, the USA; Dr J. Martin, National Institute for Biological Standards and Control, the United Kingdom; Dr T. Wu, Health Canada, Canada; and Dr H-N. Kang, World Health Organization, Switzerland, taking into consideration the comments received from the second Working Group Meeting and from Dr N. Previsani (*provided the consolidated comments of the WHO Containment Advisory Group*), World Health Organization, Switzerland.

The resulting draft document was then posted on the WHO Biologicals website for a first round of public consultation from 6 March to 4 April 2018 and comments were received from the following reviewers: Dr B.D. Akanmori, World Health Organization, Gabon; Dr P. Barbosa (*provided the consolidated comments of IFPMA and of the non-IFPMA manufacturers Intravacc, Biological E. Limited and AJ Vaccines*), Switzerland; C. Cahill (*provided the consolidated comments of sIPV manufacturers: I. Rudebeck and A. Thomas, AJ Vaccines; Dr C. Breda, Biological E. Limited; Dr I. Knott, J-B. Mayet and C. Pierret, GlaxoSmithKline Vaccines; W. Bakker and J. Boes, Intravacc; C. Cahill, N. Papic and X.B. Vinken, Janssen Vaccines; J. Hanselaer and J.M. Malby, Sanofi Pasteur*), Netherlands; Ms E. Febrina, National Agency of Drug and Food Control, Indonesia; Dr J. Fournier-Caruana, World Health Organization, Switzerland; Dr P.J. Huntly, Riskren PTE Ltd, Singapore; Dr A. Malkin (*provided the consolidated comments of the Chumakov Federal Scientific Center for Research and Development of Immune-and-Biological Products*), Russian Federation; Mr W. Meng (*provided the consolidated comments of Sinovac Biotech Co.*), China; Dr C. Milne, European Directorate for the Quality of Medicines & HealthCare, France; Dr P. Minor, London, the United Kingdom; Dr H. Shimizu (provided the consolidated comments of the sIPV Working Group in Japan), National Institute of Infectious Diseases, Japan; Mr G. Singh, Bharat Biotech International Ltd, India; and Professor Y. Yao, Institute of Medical Biology, China.

The document WHO/BS/2018.2350 was prepared by the above WHO Drafting Group, taking into consideration the comments received from the first round of public consultation as well as from the Third WHO Working Group meeting on developing WHO Guidelines on the safe production of polio vaccines held in Geneva, Switzerland, 7–8 May 2018 and attended by: Ms A. Bonhomme, Public Health Agency of Canada, Canada; Dr X. Bouwstra, Bilthoven Biologicals BV, Netherlands; Ms I.S. Budiharto, PT Bio Farma, Indonesia (*DCVMN representative*); Dr K. Chumakov, United States Food and Drug Administration, the USA; Dr R. Dhere, Serum Institute of India, India (*DCVMN representative*);

Mr S. Dong, Institute of Medical Biology, China (*DCVMN representative*); Mr M. Duchene, Janssen Vaccines, Netherlands (*IFPMA representative*); Dr M. Engelkes, National Institute for Public Health and the Environment, Netherlands; Dr S. Fakhrzadeh, Food and Drug Administration, the Islamic Republic of Iran; Dr E. Grabski, Paul-Ehrlich-Institute, Germany; Mr J. Hanselaer, Sanofi Pasteur, France (*IFPMA representative*); Dr Y. Ichimura, Ministry of Health, Labour and Welfare, Japan; Dr J. Jung, Ministry of Food and Drug Safety, Republic of Korea; Mr H. Kaghazian, Pasteur Institute of Iran, the Islamic Republic of Iran (*DCVMN representative*); Ms I. Knott, GlaxoSmithKline Vaccines, Belgium (*IFPMA representative*); Dr M. Kooijman, Institute for Translational Vaccinology, Netherlands; Mr P. Krati, Praha Vaccines, Czechia; Dr K. Mahmood, PATH, the USA; Dr A. Malkin, Chumakov Federal Scientific Center for Research and Development of Immune-and-Biological Products, Russian Federation; Dr J. Martin, National Institute for Biological Standards and Control, the United Kingdom; Mr W. Meng, Sinovac Biotech, China (*DCVMN representative*); Mr T. Okada, BIKEN, Japan; Dr K.N. Olsen, Statens Serum Institut, Denmark; Dr S. Pawar, Ministry of Health and Family Welfare, India; Dr V. Pithon, Agence nationale de sécurité du médicament et des produits de santé, France; Mr M. Polan, Praha Vaccines, Czechia; Dr M. Reers, Biological E. Limited, India (*DCVMN representative*); Ms I. Rudebeck, AJ Vaccines, Denmark; Dr R.C. Sanders, the United Kingdom; Mr T. Satou, Takeda Vaccines, Japan (*IFPMA representative*); Mr G. Singh, Bharat Biotech, India (*DCVMN representative*); Dr A. Sinyugina, Chumakov Federal Scientific Center for Research and Development of Immune-and-Biological Products, Russian Federation; Mr Y. Someya, National Institute of Infectious Diseases, Japan; Dr T. Tanimoto, BIKEN, Japan; Dr C.R. Villumsen, Ministry of Health, Denmark; Dr T. Wu, Health Canada, Canada; Ms W. Wulandari, National Agency of Drug and Food Control, Indonesia; and Dr M. Eisenhawer, Dr J. Fournier-Caruana, Mr M. Janssen, Dr H-N. Kang, Dr I. Knezevic and Dr N. Previsani, World Health Organization, Switzerland.

The document WHO/BS/2018.2350 was then posted on the WHO Biologicals website for a second round of public consultation from 25 July to 28 September 2018 and comments were received from the following reviewers: Dr P. Barbosa (*provided the consolidated comments of IFPMA*), Dr X. Bouwstra-Vinken, Bilthoven Biologicals BV, Netherlands; Dr J. Fournier-Caruana, World Health Organization, Switzerland; Mr N. Godden, WHO Containment Advisory Group; Dr V. Halkjaer-Knudsen, WHO Containment Advisory Group; Dr P.J. Huntly, Riskren PTE Ltd, Singapore; Dr M. Janssen, World Health Organization, Switzerland; Dr A.K. Tahlan and Dr R.P. Roy, Central Research Institute, India; Mr M. Polan, Praha Vaccines, Czechia; Mr G. Singh, Bharat Biotech, India; Dr J. Southern, Consultant, South Africa.

Further changes were subsequently made to document WHO/BS/ 2018.2350 by the WHO Expert Committee on Biological Standardization.

References

1. Guidelines for the safe production and quality control of inactivated poliomyelitis vaccine manufactured from wild polioviruses (Addendum, 2003, to the Recommendations for the production and quality control of poliomyelitis vaccine (inactivated)). In: WHO Expert Committee on Biological Standardization: fifty-third report. Geneva: World Health Organization; 2004: Annex 2 (WHO Technical Report Series, No.926; http://www.who.int/biologicals/publications/trs/areas/vaccines/polio/Annex%202%20%2865-89%29TRS926Polio2003.pdf, accessed 9 June 2018).

2. Recommendations for the production and control of poliomyelitis vaccine (inactivated). Replacement of Requirements for poliomyelitis vaccine (inactivated) of WHO Technical Report Series, No. 673; and Annex 4 of WHO Technical Report Series, No. 745. In: WHO Expert Committee on Biological Standardization: fifty-first report. Geneva: World Health Organization; 2002: Annex 2 (WHO Technical Report Series, No. 910; http://www.who.int/biologicals/publications/trs/areas/vaccines/polio/WHO_TRS_910_Annex2_polioinactivated.pdf, accessed 9 June 2018).

3. Recommendations to assure the quality, safety and efficacy of poliomyelitis vaccines (inactivated). Replacement of Annex 2 of WHO Technical Report Series, No. 910. In: WHO Expert Committee on Biological Standardization: sixty-fifth report. Geneva: World Health Organization; 2015: Annex 3 (WHO Technical Report Series, No. 993; http://www.who.int/biologicals/vaccines/Annex3_IPV_Recommendations_eng.pdf?ua=1, accessed 9 June 2018).

4. Recommendations to assure the quality, safety and efficacy of poliomyelitis vaccines (oral, live, attenuated). Replacement of Annex 1 of WHO Technical Report Series, No. 904; and Addendum to Annex 1 of WHO Technical Report Series, No. 910. In: WHO Expert Committee on Biological Standardization: sixty-third report. Geneva: World Health Organization; 2014: Annex 2 (WHO Technical Report Series, No. 980; http://www.who.int/biologicals/vaccines/OPV_Recommendations_TRS_980_Annex_2.pdf?ua=1, accessed 9 June 2018).

5. WHO good manufacturing practices for pharmaceutical products: main principles. Replacement of Annex 3 of WHO Technical Report Series, No. 961. In: WHO Expert Committee on Specifications for Pharmaceutical Preparations: forty-eighth report. Geneva: World Health Organization; 2014: Annex 2 (WHO Technical Report Series, No. 986; http://www.who.int/medicines/areas/quality_safety/quality_assurance/TRS986annex2.pdf?ua=1, accessed 9 June 2018).

6. WHO good manufacturing practices for biological products. Replacement of Annex 1 of WHO Technical Report Series, No. 822. In: WHO Expert Committee on Biological Standardization: sixty-sixth report. Geneva: World Health Organization; 2016: Annex 2 (WHO Technical Report Series, No. 999; http://www.who.int/biologicals/areas/vaccines/Annex_2_WHO_Good_manufacturing_practices_for_biological_products.pdf?ua=1, accessed 9 June 2018).

7. WHO Global Action Plan to minimize poliovirus facility-associated risk after type-specific eradication of wild polioviruses and sequential cessation of oral polio vaccine use. GAPIII. Geneva: World Health Organization; 2015 (http://polioeradication.org/wp-content/uploads/2016/12/GAPIII_2014.pdf, accessed 9 June 2018).

8. Revision of Guidelines on the safe production and quality control of inactivated poliomyelitis vaccines manufactured from wild polioviruses. In: WHO Expert Committee on Biological Standardization: sixty-sixth report. Geneva: World Health Organization; 2016: 41–2 (WHO Technical Report Series, No. 999: 41–2; http://apps.who.int/iris/bitstream/10665/208900/1/9789240695634-eng.pdf?ua=1, accessed 9 June 2018).

9. Revision of WHO Guidelines for the safe production and quality control of inactivated poliomyelitis vaccines manufactured from wild polioviruses. In: WHO Expert Committee on Biological Standardization: sixty-seventh report. Geneva: World Health Organization; 2017 (WHO Technical Report Series, No. 1004: 43–4; http://apps.who.int/iris/bitstream/10665/255657/1/9789241210133-eng.pdf?ua=1, accessed 9 June 2018).

10. Laboratory biosafety manual. Third edition. Geneva: World Health Organization; 2004 (http://www.who.int/csr/resources/publications/biosafety/Biosafety7.pdf?ua=1, accessed 9 June 2018).

11. Biorisk management. Laboratory biosecurity guidance. Geneva: World Health Organization; 2006 (http://www.who.int/csr/resources/publications/biosafety/WHO_CDS_EPR_2006_6.pdf, accessed 9 June 2018).

12. Report of the third teleconference of the Containment Advisory Group (CAG TC3) on novel oral poliomyelitis type 2 candidate vaccines and S19-poliovirus type 2 strains, 7 June 2018 (http://polioeradication.org/wp-content/uploads/2018/09/CAG_TC3_June_2018_EN_Final.pdf, accessed 28 November 2018).

13. GAPIII Containment Certification Scheme. Geneva: World Health Organization; 2017 (http://polioeradication.org/wp-content/uploads/2017/03/CCS_19022017-EN.pdf, accessed 9 June 2018).

14. Resolution WHA41.28. Global eradication of poliomyelitis by the year 2000. Forty-first World Health Assembly, Geneva, 2–13 May 1988. Geneva: World Health Organization; 1988 (http://www.who.int/ihr/polioresolution4128en.pdf, accessed 9 June 2018).

15. Meeting of the Strategic Advisory Group of Experts on Immunization, April 2017 – conclusions and recommendations. Wkly Epidemiol Rec. No 22, 2 June 2017;92:301–20 (http://apps.who.int/iris/bitstream/10665/255611/1/WER9222.pdf?ua=1, accessed 9 June 2018).

16. Global polio eradication: progress towards containment of poliovirus type 2, worldwide 2017. Wkly Epidemiol Rec. No 25, 23 June 2017;92:350–6 (http://apps.who.int/iris/bitstream/handle/10665/255748/WER9225.pdf?sequence=1, accessed 9 June 2018).

17. Technical Guidance: mOPV2 vaccine management, monitoring, removal and validation. Geneva: World Health Organization for the Global Polio Eradication Initiative; 2016 (http://polioeradication.org/wp-content/uploads/2016/11/Technical-guidance-mOPV2-management-monitoring-removal-and-validation_Oct2016_EN.pdf, accessed 28 November 2018).

18. Polio Eradication & Endgame Strategic Plan 2013–2018. Geneva: World Health Organization for the Global Polio Eradication Initiative; 2013 (http://polioeradication.org/wp-content/uploads/2016/07/PEESP_EN_A4.pdf, accessed 9 June 2018).

19. Sabin AB, Boulger LR. History of Sabin attenuated poliovirus oral live vaccine strains. J Biol Stand. 1973;1(2):115–8 (abstract: https://www.sciencedirect.com/science/article/pii/0092115773900486, accessed 9 June 2018).

20. Katz M, Plotkin SA. Minimal infective dose of attenuated poliovirus for man. Am J Public Health Nations Health. 1967;57(10):1837–40 (https://www.ncbi.nlm.nih.gov/pmc/articles/PMC1227778/pdf/amjphnation00078-0125.pdf, accessed 9 June 2018).

21. Minor TE, Allen CI, Tsiatis AA, Nelson DB, D'Alessio DJ. Human infective dose determinations for oral poliovirus type 1 vaccine in infants. J Clin Microbiol. 1981;13(2):388–9 (https://www.ncbi.nlm.nih.gov/pmc/articles/PMC273794/pdf/jcm00163-0172.pdf, accessed 9 June 2018).

22. Duizer E, Ruijs WL, van der Weijden CP, Timen A. Response to a wild poliovirus type 2 (WPV2)-shedding event following accidental exposure to WPV2, the Netherlands, April 2017. Euro Surveill. 2017;22(21):30542 (https://www.eurosurveillance.org/content/10.2807/1560-7917.ES.2017.22.21.30542, accessed 9 June 2018).

23. Duizer E, Rutjes S, de Roda Husman AM, Schijven J. Risk assessment, risk management and risk-based monitoring following a reported accidental release of poliovirus in Belgium, September to November 2014. Euro Surveill. 2016;21(11):30169 (https://www.eurosurveillance.org/content/10.2807/1560-7917.ES.2016.21.11.30169, accessed 9 June 2018).

24. Mulders MN, Reimerink JHJ, Koopmans MP, van Loon AM, van der Avoort HGAM. Genetic analysis of wild-type poliovirus importation into the Netherlands (1979–1995). J Infect Dis. 1997;176(3):617–24 (https://www.researchgate.net/publication/13930487_Genetic_analysis_of_wild-type_poliovirus_importation_into_The_Netherlands_1979-1995, accessed 10 June 2018).

25. Tyler R, Ayliffe GAJ, Bradley C. Virucidal activity of disinfectants: studies with the poliovirus. J Hosp Infect. 1990;15(4):339–45 (abstract: https://www.sciencedirect.com/science/article/pii/019567019090090B, accessed 10 June 2018).

26. Dowdle WR, Birmingham ME. The biologic principles of poliovirus eradication. J Infect Dis. 1997;175(Suppl 1):S286–92 (abstract: https://www.researchgate.net/publication/14015093_The_Biologic_Principles_of_Poliovirus_Eradication, accessed 10 June 2018).

27. Ionidis G, Hübscher J, Jack T, Becker B, Bischoff B, Todt D et al. Development and virucidal activity of a novel alcohol-based hand disinfectant supplemented with urea and citric acid. BMC Infect Dis. 2016;16:77 (https://bmcinfectdis.biomedcentral.com/articles/10.1186/s12879-016-1410-9, accessed 10 June 2018).

28. Report of the second meeting of the Containment Advisory Group (CAG), Geneva, Switzerland, 28–30 November 2017 (http://polioeradication.org/wp-content/uploads/2018/02/poliovirus-containment-advisory-group-meeting-20171130.pdf, accessed 10 June 2018).

29. Report of the first teleconference of the Containment Advisory Group (CAG TC1) on showers, 25 January 2018 (http://polioeradication.org/wp-content/uploads/2018/04/poliovirus-containment-advisory-group-teleconference-20180125-en.pdf, accessed 28 November 2018).

30. Report of the second teleconference of the Containment Advisory Group (CAG TC2) on novel poliovirus strains, 8 March 2018 (http://polioeradication.org/wp-content/uploads/2018/05/containment-advisory-group-novel-poliovirus-strains-8-march-2018-20180518.pdf, accessed 28 November 2018).

31. WHO good manufacturing practices for pharmaceutical products containing hazardous substances. In: WHO Expert Committee on Specifications for Pharmaceutical Preparations: forty-fourth report. Geneva: World Health Organization; 2010: Annex 3 (WHO Technical Report Series, No. 957; http://www.who.int/medicines/areas/quality_safety/quality_assurance/GMPPharmaceuticalProductsCcontainingHhazardousSubstancesTRS957Annex3.pdf, accessed 10 June 2018).

32. Guidelines on heating, ventilation and air-conditioning systems for non-sterile pharmaceutical products. In: WHO Expert Committee on Specifications for Pharmaceutical Preparations: fifty-second report. Geneva: World Health Organization; 2018: Annex 8 (WHO Technical Report Series, No. 1010; http://apps.who.int/iris/bitstream/handle/10665/272452/9789241210195-eng.pdf, accessed 28 November 2018).

33. WHO good manufacturing practices: water for pharmaceutical use. Replacement of Annex 3 of WHO Technical Report Series, No. 929. In: WHO Expert Committee on Specifications for Pharmaceutical Preparations: forty-sixth report. Geneva: World Health Organization; 2012: Annex 2 (WHO Technical Report Series, No. 970; http://www.who.int/medicines/areas/quality_safety/quality_assurance/GMPWatePharmaceuticalUseTRS970Annex2.pdf?ua=1, accessed 10 June 2018).

34.	Standard Operating Procedure. Neurovirulence test of types 1, 2 or 3 live attenuated poliomyelitis vaccines (oral) in monkeys. Geneva: World Health Organization; 2012 (http://www.who.int/biologicals/vaccines/MNVT_SOP_Final_09112012.pdf?ua=1, accessed 10 June 2018).

35.	Standard Operating Procedure. Neurovirulence test of types 1, 2 or 3 live attenuated poliomyelitis vaccines (oral) in transgenic mice susceptible to poliovirus. Geneva: World Health Organization; 2015 (http://www.who.int/biologicals/vaccines/POLIO_SOP_TgmNVT_SOPv7_30_June2015_CLEAN2.pdf?ua=1, accessed 10 June 2018).

36.	Standard Operating Procedure. Mutant analysis by PCR and restriction enzyme cleavage (MAPREC) for oral poliovirus (Sabin) vaccine types 1, 2 or 3. Geneva: World Health Organization; 2012 (http://www.who.int/biologicals/vaccines/MAPREC_SOP_Final_09112012.pdf?ua=1, accessed 10 June 2018).

37.	Neverov A, Chumakov K. Massively parallel sequencing for monitoring genetic consistency and quality control of live viral vaccines. Proc Natl Acad Sci U S A. 2010;107(46):20063–8 (http://www.pnas.org/content/pnas/107/46/20063.full.pdf, accessed 10 June 2018).

Annex 5

Biological substances: WHO International Standards, Reference Reagents and Reference Panels

The provision of global measurement standards is a core normative WHO activity. WHO reference materials are widely used by manufacturers, regulatory authorities and academic researchers in the development and evaluation of biological products. The timely development of new reference materials is crucial in harnessing the benefits of scientific advances in new biologicals and in vitro diagnosis. At the same time, management of the existing inventory of reference preparations requires an active and carefully planned programme of work to replace established materials before existing stocks are exhausted.

The considerations and guiding principles used to assign priorities and develop the programme of work in this area have previously been set out as WHO Recommendations.[18] In order to facilitate and improve transparency in the priority-setting process, a simple tool was developed as Appendix 1 of these WHO Recommendations. This tool describes the key considerations taken into account when assigning priorities, and allows stakeholders to review and comment on any new proposals being considered for endorsement by the WHO Expert Committee on Biological Standardization.

A list of current WHO International Standards, Reference Reagents and Reference Panels for biological substances is available at: http://www.who.int/biologicals.

At its meeting held on 29 October to 2 November 2018, the WHO Expert Committee on Biological Standardization made the changes shown below to the previous list. Each of the preparations shown in this table should be used in accordance with their instructions for use (IFU).

---

[18] Recommendations for the preparation, characterization and establishment of international and other biological reference standards (revised 2004). In: WHO Expert Committee on Biological Standardization: fifty-fifth report. Geneva: World Health Organization; 2006: Annex 2 (WHO Technical Report Series, No. 932; http://www.who.int/immunization_standards/vaccine_reference_preparations/TRS932Annex%202_Inter%20_biol%20ef%20standards%20rev2004.pdf?ua=1, accessed 27 March 2018).

Additions[19]

Preparation	Unitage	Status
Antibiotics		
Erythromycin*	925 IU/mg	Third WHO International Standard
Blood products and related substances		
Blood coagulation factor V (plasma, human)	FV:C = 0.72 IU/ampoule FV:Ag = 0.75 IU/ampoule	Second WHO International Standard
Anti-D immunoglobulin (human)	297 IU/ampoule	Third WHO International Standard
In vitro diagnostics		
CD4+ T-cells (human)	[no assigned units]	First WHO International Reference Reagent
HIV-1 p24 antigen	[no assigned units]	First WHO International Reference Panel
HIV-2 p26 antigen	[no assigned units]	First WHO International Reference Reagent
von Willebrand factor (plasma) binding to recombinant glycoprotein Ib	VWF:GPIbM = 0.87 u/ampoule VWF:GPIbR = 0.87 u/ampoule	First WHO International Reference Reagent
Prostate specific antigen (human) (free)	0.53 µg/ampoule	Second WHO International Standard
Prostate specific antigen (human) (total: PSA-ACT + free PSA)	0.50 µg/ampoule	Second WHO International Standard
HIV-2 RNA for NAT-based assays	1.44×10^5 IU/vial	Second WHO International Standard
Adenovirus DNA for NAT-based assays	2.0×10^8 IU/vial	First WHO International Standard

---

[19] Unless otherwise indicated, all materials are held and distributed by the National Institute for Biological Standards and Control, Potters Bar, Herts, EN6 3QG, the United Kingdom. Materials identified by an * in the above list are held and distributed by the European Directorate for the Quality of Medicines & Healthcare, Strasbourg 67081, France.

Preparation	Unitage	Status
Standards for use in public health emergencies		
Anti-Asian lineage Zika virus antibody (human)	250 IU/ampoule	First WHO International Standard
Vaccines and related substances		
MRC-5 cells	[no assigned units]	Second WHO International Reference Cell Bank
Rabies vaccine	8.9 IU/ampoule (NIH mouse potency test) 2.5 IU/ampoule (ELISA for glycoprotein) 2.9 IU/ampoule (SRD for glycoprotein)	Seventh WHO International Standard
Sabin inactivated poliomyelitis vaccine	100 Sabin D-Ag Unit (SDU)/ml for poliovirus type 1 100 SDU/ml for poliovirus type 2 100 SDU/ml for poliovirus type 3	First WHO International Standard